More praise for
STOLEN TOMORROWS

"Steven Levenkron hits the core of women's childhood sexual abuse with vivid human portrayals, fleshing out a compassionate and practical guide that puts human faces on this overwhelming problem."

—Lynn Ponton, MD, author of *The Romance of Risk: Why Teenagers Do the Things They Do* and *The Sex Lives of Teenagers: Revealing the Secret World of Adolescent Boys and Girls*

"*Stolen Tomorrows* is a book for every clinician and those not familiar with the subtle yet powerful impact of sexual abuse. Levenkron shows how sexual trauma can impact relationships, addictions, belief systems, and the physiological responses the body imprints from the experience. Well done!"

—Melissa Bradley, MS, NCC, Board Certified Expert in Traumatic Stress

"Steven Levenkron has once again written a wonderful book. . . . It offers realistic hope for us all, especially for the many untreated women worldwide whose lives have been profoundly diminished by their experience of childhood sexual abuse."

—Michael Kenin, MD, New York University School of Medicine

"As a clinician who has studied and treated sexual abuse survivors for many years, I was thrilled to read this comprehensive, sensitive, and hopeful book. . . . This is a must-read for all professionals who treat sexual abuse survivors as well as for the patients themselves. . . . The combination of important research information and sensitive case studies provides the reader with a realistic yet optimistic view of the possibility of emerging from the shadows of trauma."

—Karen Binder-Brynes, PhD, clinical instructor of psychiatry, Mt. Sinai School of Medicine

STOLEN
TOMORROWS

Understanding and Treating

Women's Childhood

Sexual Abuse

STEVEN LEVENKRON

WITH ABBY LEVENKRON

W. W. NORTON & COMPANY

NEW YORK   LONDON

For information about permission to reproduce selections from this book,
write to Permissions, W. W. Norton & Company, Inc.
500 Fifth Avenue, New York, NY 10110

Manufacturing by RR Donnelley, Harrisonburg
Book design by JAM Design
Production manager: Andrew Marasia

Library of Congress Cataloging-in-Publication Data

Levenkron, Steven, 1941–
Stolen tomorrows : understanding and treating women's childhood
sexual abuse / Steven Levenkron, with Abby Levenkron. — 1st ed.
p. cm.
Includes bibliographical references and index.
ISBN-13: 978-0-393-06086-7 (hardcover)
ISBN-10: 0-393-06086-1 (hardcover)
1. Adult child sexual abuse victims—Psychology. 2. Adult child sexual abuse victims—
Treatment. 3. Psychotherapy. I. Levenkron, Abby. II. Title.
RC569.5.A28L48 2007
616.85'83690651—dc22
2006035743

ISBN 978-0-393-33201-8 pbk.

W. W. Norton & Company, Inc.
500 Fifth Avenue, New York, N.Y. 10110
www.wwnorton.com

W. W. Norton & Company Ltd.
Castle House, 75/76 Wells Street, London W1T 3QT

1 2 3 4 5 6 7 8 9 0

This book is dedicated to

the recovery of all the women

who have survived

childhood sexual abuse

Contents

PART THREE: Understanding Stolen Tomorrows

PART FOUR: Recovering Stolen Tomorrows

Toxic Water, Stunted Tree: An Introduction to Childhood Sexual Abuse

If you plant a young tree beside an underground stream of toxic water, its roots will grow down until they reach that water. Every aspect of the tree's growth, from roots to leaves, will be shaped by the contaminated water: the trunk will be stunted, the bark distorted, and finally the tree may bear peculiar leaves and diseased fruit. We may all notice this tree, its leaves and fruit, but how many of us would question the water that contaminated the soil wherein it grew?

If, before puberty, a girl is raped or sexually touched, and in the process

- made to feel pain and terror

- caused to feel helpless and vulnerable to destruction

- shattered and made to flee consciousness

then her future life choices have been changed and her ability to make those choices has been altered—In short, her tomorrows have been stolen.

In this book we seek to explain the adulthood outcomes of childhood sexual abuse and the damage it wreaks. We will examine what was going on "beneath the surface" during the child's growing years and how these experiences have affected and shaped her growth. As recounted through therapy sessions, we will see the toxic effects of abuse and the survivor's thoughts about herself in reaction to the abuse as she works to understand her personality, her behaviors, her relationships, and her lifestyle. Returning to our opening metaphor, we will observe the peculiar fruit of childhood sexual abuse in terms of how the damage developed invisibly, as it does beneath the opaque bark of a growing tree fed by toxic waters.

Numerous books have been written about childhood sexual abuse. Some of these are statistical studies of large populations; some are case histories of treatment, or individual reports of personal experiences. In this book, which can be characterized as a psychotherapist's notebook, we will discuss different cases of sexual abuse in which young girls, ages one to twelve, were the victims. More important than the graphic details of the abuse are the different settings: the nature of the girl's relationship to her abuser (father, uncle, brother, grandfather, friend of the family, authority figure in the community, or stranger), the duration or number of assaults, the length of time they continued (months to years), and how long the child carried her secret before getting help. Additional factors include the character and attitude of the perpetrator and how these alter the victim's personality as she tries to interpret the meaning of the event, her role in the event, and her judgment of herself.

Her reaction to these childhood experiences will affect her development with regard to everything from psychological disorders, to personality characteristics, to lifestyle. All of these outward effects reflect her way of coping with her feelings during the abusive period of her life.

After examining the damage that results from years of adapting to her abuse, we will describe and discuss means of recovery, including forms of psychotherapy, medication, caring friends, support groups, and family involvement.

PREVALENCE OF ABUSE

We must be concerned with these behaviors by older persons toward children because of the devastating and often permanent harm that they cause through adolescence and adulthood, when most abuse survivors come for treatment. It is important to note that in the United States, the prevalence of childhood sexual abuse, as documented by congressional findings, the National Institute of Mental Health, and other reputable researchers including the Child Welfare Information Gateway, a part of the U.S. Department of Health and Human Services, varies from 15 to 30 percent.[1]

There have been many studies on the prevalence of child sexual abuse. The statistics can be confusing because "unwanted sexual contact including rape" has been estimated to be from 12 to 36 percent in the United States.[2] However, if we assume from these estimates an average of approximately 20 percent, then the personalities of about one in five females have been affected by this kind of experience. This is a significant portion of the population who deserve help—compassion, support, and therapy.

SOME ASSUMPTIONS MADE IN THIS BOOK

The reader may wonder about my exclusive use of the pronoun "she" throughout this book, as well as the absence of discussion about male childhood sexual abuse. My psychotherapy practice since the 1978 publication of *The Best Little Girl in the World* became, and has remained, almost exclusively female. The reason this book focuses on female childhood sexual abuse is that all my abused patients are female.

All of the perpetrators presented here are males. In my years of doing long-term individual psychotherapy with dozens of women who were sexually abused as children, the perpetrators have all been males. This is not to say that female perpetrators abusing children do not exist. We do not know the precise ratio of male perpetrators to female perpetrators, but it is generally accepted that the large majority are males.

PART ONE

■

THEN AND NOW

1

The Sexually Abused Child as an Adult

Childhood sexual abuse derails normal personality development, creating a variety of alternative outcomes and causing behaviors to develop that will further damage the victim. The moment a child is abused, with no one to tell about it, is the moment she understands there is no one to protect her. She will develop a variety of defenses, real and imaginary, to provide a sense of safety, or she will attempt to produce a feeling of insensitivity and emotional numbness to whatever is happening to her.

The ways she devises to protect herself may go unnoticed for years. When they emerge for others around her to witness, these defenses may seem bizarre or foolish to some, immoral to others. It is important to remember that these mechanisms developed and evolved years before they emerged in the child's conscious mind. The child who was repeatedly traumatized had no hope that the assaultive behavior would ever end, and no context within which to understand it. As we look at the case histories of the women in Part Two, we will see how each devised her own concepts for understanding the episodes she suffered through and how she acted on these concepts.

When a child feels overpowered, helpless, and damaged, she will, most likely, blame herself. If she can develop a perspective that excludes blaming herself, which is rare, she may suffer less damage. Or, as she grows up, she may learn how to hurt others that resemble her assaulter or may adopt the identity and behavior of her assaulter. Later chapters will show how the child's personality follows these separate and different directions, step by step, and explain what can be done in therapy to direct her toward making choices in her own best interests, free from fear and conflict. This will be the goal of therapy when she seeks professional help.

THE CASE HISTORIES: A PREVIEW

At the beginning of treatment the therapist knows very little of the patient's history—perhaps only what we call the *presenting problem*, the reason she was referred to therapy by a doctor, a loved one, a friend or sought out therapy herself. Here in brief are some of the cases presented in this book; "Then" refers to the time the abuse began, while "Now" refers to the woman's situation the day treatment started and describes recent behaviors and events that comprise the presenting problem.

Cassie   **Then:** Cassie was a seven-year-old compliant daughter. Her mother was a full-time housewife, and her father, a general surgeon, was a pillar of the community. From ages seven to eleven, Cassie was raped at night in her bed by her father.

   Now: Cassie is a fifty-two-year-old mother and wife who spent dozens of years cheating on her husband while raising their daughter. She came to me for help dealing with her behavioral problems, which had led to neglecting her daughter. Cassie always has a terrified look on her face.

Olivia   **Then:** Olivia was a shy, five-year-old girl learning penmanship in the first grade, living with her mother and stepfather, a wealthy businessman. He nightly molested her while telling her it was good for her. This went on for five years.

Now: She is married, thirty-two, and incapable of being sexually aroused. Her husband is divorcing her. They have two children.

Adrienne   Then: Adrienne was a happy five-year-old until her uncle began molesting her, under water, while swimming at the southern beach where both families lived. In all her childhood photos she is frowning.

Now: Adrienne, at twenty, dates boys who exploit her, drinks to excess, and uses combinations of drugs to attempt to sleep at night. She was raped as a teen, has had anorexia for two years, dropped out of college, and is generally depressed. (*Anorexia nervosa*, often simply called anorexia, is an eating disorder in which the person drastically restricts her food intake, becoming dangerously thin out of a distorted fear of becoming fat. Untreated, the person may die of starvation.)

Audrey   Then: Audrey remembers first being molested on a changing table when she was an infant and later, as a child aged five to eight, by her father. She remembers being aroused and experiencing what she later learned was an orgasm. She felt a peculiar attachment to her father that she did not understand.

Now: Audrey dropped out of high school when she was sixteen. She had no girl friends and turned to boys for friendship and sex. She went through a period of anorexia nervosa. She came to treatment at age twenty-four. She uses cocaine and marijuana, and drinks alcohol to excess, sometimes in combination. She cannot keep a regular job and frequently becomes verbally and physically enraged at others.

Jen   Then: Jen represents an unusual case in that what she experienced was not intentionally perpetrated abuse. She was diagnosed as suffering from urinary reflux, which causes urine to back up to the kidneys, leading to frequent kidney infections. Unchecked this would eventually damage her kidneys; requiring surgery. In an attempt to avoid surgery, the urologist catheterized Jen from ages seven to eleven, on a monthly basis for several hours. She found this treatment embarrassing, terrifying, and painful—in short, she experienced it as sexual assault. At eleven, Jen had to undergo the deferred surgery anyway.

Now: At nineteen, Jen cuts herself and dresses seductively. In her relationships with men, she is dependent and they treat her sadistically. She is a compulsive shopper, and despite the unlimited financial resources of her family, she also shoplifts, for which she has been arrested once. She dissociates (losing conscious awareness of her surroundings) for hours at a time, suffers from *derealization* (feeling unable to be present in the moment or current situation), and blacks out. She crashed the family car during one such episode. Her feelings about people change mercurially from liking them to disliking them.

June   **Then:** From five to twelve years of age, June was molested by her brother. In addition, he drilled holes in her bathroom wall to spy on her. The molestation was done in a seductive manner, and she experienced arousal during these episodes. At other times he would physically abuse her, tie her up, and hit her. Her brother's treatment of her was inconsistent: he would praise her when she brought home good grades.

Now: June came to treatment for anorexia at age twenty-seven. She explained she is only attracted to abusive men, some of whom exploit her financially. She is in the process of divorcing her husband. Kind men do not arouse her sexually. At our second session she tells me she fears I will become bored with her, will dislike her, will decide not to treat her, and will abuse her. (Despite her fears, she stays in treatment continuously for seven years.)

Now that we have a sampling of some of the women whose stories will be given more fully later on, let's examine childhood sexual abuse more generally.

SEXUAL ABUSE: DEFINITIONS AND KEY INDICATORS

Sexual abuse is defined broadly as one person taking advantage of another through sexual contact or behavior that is unwanted by the recipient, causing that person emotional, psychological, and usually physical pain. By extension, then, *childhood sexual abuse* is defined by a relationship involving physical acts of violation committed by a person or persons who are older and/or more powerful than the child.

When arousal occurs as a result of sexual contact, the recipient may experience additional confusion about the definition of "unwanted" sexual behavior and feel ashamed: she may assume that being aroused makes her complicit in the abusive sex acts. Whether or not arousal occurs, a child who has suffered sexual abuse has been victimized and will experience serious, painful consequences.

How does a child know she has been abused? She is aware that she has been violated, although she lacks the vocabulary to express this. Feeling dishonored, sullied, or debased makes her feel less valuable than before, in particular, less valuable than those around her.

The experience is similar to being ostracized, a word with a long history. During the time of the Greek empire, when a nobleman was convicted of disgraceful behavior, he would be handed a piece of a broken clay pot. This jagged piece of clay was called *ostracon* and meant that he and his family were to be exiled for a period of ten years. He then often refused food and drink until he died. Ostracism (which still occurs in a number of groups and cultures) was and is a social process. Child abuse is not. Yet a person—child or adult—may infer a kind of implied ostracism or implied disgrace as the result of sexual abuse.

Many women who were molested as children speak about "feeling dirty." They mean that part of their body is contaminated, immoral, and repulsive. A girl who experiences an invasion or use of her body against her will comes to this conclusion by observing the demeanor of the perpetrator. When his expressed attitude is aggressive, derisive, mocking, gloating, delighted, or indifferent to her protests, no matter how subtle or assertive, she realizes she has been violated. It does not take a complex vocabulary, or even verbal thought, for her to understand her state of debasement.

Implicit in this terrifying experience is the child's sense of helplessness to stop the episode while it's occurring or to stop it from recurring in the future. Toward this end, the child may develop superstitious thinking and beliefs about behaviors she hopes will stop or minimize future episodes of abuse. When she acts on her "magical thinking" others noticing these strange behaviors may criticize her or send her for psychotherapy. The following descriptions are typical behaviors she may develop (though this is not a complete list):

- Beginning at age eleven (or earlier), she wants other girls or boys to look at or touch her chest, breasts (if they've begun to develop), labia, or anus.

- She begins drinking alcohol by age fourteen, thirteen, or even younger, and becomes dependent on it to such an extent as to be considered an alcoholic.

- She abuses other substances, either prescription drugs (tranquilizers or sleeping pills) or street drugs (such as cocaine, heroine, or methamphetamines) on a regular basis. This suggests she is *self-medicating*, using drugs to "manage" her trauma on a daily basis.

- She begins to self-mutilate, cutting or burning herself in secret.

- During her teens she seeks out relationships with abusive boys and/or girls.

- She speaks openly about being ugly, dirty, or a bad person.

- She shows signs of withdrawal, depression, and social isolation.

- She becomes a self-mutilator.

- She develops an eating disorder (anorexia nervosa and/or bulimia) or obsessive-compulsive disorder.

- She becomes a compulsive overeater.

- By her late teens she shows no interest in boys.

- She dresses in men's clothes or in clothes that conceal her female curves.

- She dresses seductively with inappropriate degrees of exposure, and acts out with aggressive sexual promiscuity.

- She consistently becomes anxious in the presence of one member of the family, or avoids that person.

None of these behaviors by themselves indicate a history of childhood sexual abuse, but a history of several or many of them requires considering that as a possibility.

Flashbacks, dreams, and memories   Key indicators of child molestation and rape also include flashbacks to actual events, and disturbing, recurrent dreams about similar events. A *flashback* is a painfully vivid reexperiencing of an event so traumatic that it has no boundaries in time. It differs from ordinary memory because it not only involves thoughts and feelings but bodily reactions as well, including changes in heart rhythm, muscle contractions, perspiration, and blood pressure. Flashbacks may be provoked by something seen or heard that acts as a reminder; they may also occur randomly, with no external stimuli.

"Abuse dreams" could more accurately be called nightmares, in which the victim is continuously pursued by a menacing figure. She generally wakes up before being caught, much as other individuals awake before they come to harm in their dreams. The hallmark of the molestation dream is the persistent repetition of this theme of pursuit and intense fear.

Many individuals in their late teens or older have forgotten their childhood abuse. One patient, for example, did not remember the four childhood years she was raped by her father until she was forty-eight years old. There are several reasons for this selective amnesia, employed to protect the child emotionally at the time of the assaults. These reasons will be presented in the full context of each individual's case study in Part Two.

Other adult survivors remember their childhood abuse, but they are so intensely ashamed of these experiences that, unless they have already discussed it with someone else, they will deny it happened if a therapist asks about it prematurely, that is before developing a strong therapeutic alliance that will allow the patient to feel secure and trusting in therapy.

Defense mechanisms and other symptoms   While the behaviors listed earlier in the chapter, when seen in clusters, might indicate child abuse, it is the thoughts, mental explanations, mental strategies, and ways the growing child defines herself and her value as a person as a result of being abused that will create and influence her personality development, lifestyle, and relationships with others.

The first reaction a girl has after being molested or raped is shock and bewilderment. After trying to understand if she did anything to provoke the assault, her next task is to develop a plan to prevent it from happening again. If the perpetrator is her father, she may try to be so well behaved that he won't "get mad at her" and do it again; at this early point she may assume the assault is punishment for displeasing him. If the perpetrator is an older brother, an uncle, or a family friend, she will try to avoid him as much as possible. The closer the perpetrator is to her the more difficult avoidance becomes. If he lives in her house, visits frequently, or baby-sits for her, it is almost impossible. When avoidance is not feasible, she may resort to superstition, developing private rituals, thoughts, or a solitary monologue in an attempt to prevent future occurrences.

When the abuse happens again anyway, she becomes despairing of rescue. Neither preventive behavior nor any kind of thoughts (magical or otherwise) can stop the recurrence of abuse, so she develops ways to tolerate the intolerable. Initially, she may dissociate. *Dissociation*, believed to be a coping mechanism, occurs when the mind needs to protect itself from an overwhelmingly painful experience. Some patients describe this as "going away," a trance-like state that minimizes awareness of what is happening to their bodies and who they are with. It is as if the patient has mentally disappeared, leaving her body behind.

If the abuse is repeated—or worse, is chronic—she will try to create a context within which to view it. Because of her young age she does not have the words or ideas to explain what is happening, either to herself or anyone else. But even more critical to her problem of interpreting the abuse is that her concept of blame has not yet developed enough to assign the cause of her abuse to someone else besides herself. To do so would require a sense of self that is strong enough to contend with a person who is usually older, possibly an authority figure. A child can only perceive that for some mysterious reason, she has brought this pain, terror, and harm upon herself. This is the beginning of self-blame, which functions as a defense mechanism because it lessens her feeling of complete helplessness. Nevertheless, her self-blame will have a negative impact on her self-esteem and may evolve into self-hatred as her identity develops.

Magical thinking, dissociation, and self-blame are childhood adaptations. Later, usually in adolescence, she will add others. She may develop a behavioral disorder such as *cutting* (self-mutilation) or anorexia nervosa. She may also blame the part of her body that attracts the abuser. Her hope here is to make her body less attractive to any subsequent would-be abuser. Both anorexia and cutting thus also demonstrate a conflict with the young woman's sense of femininity. A visible aspect of anorexia is the receding of developing breasts, thighs, hips, and buttocks. Self-mutilation is an attack on the skin, generally regarded as a signifying feature of feminine beauty. These behaviors can result from either a conscious or unconscious decision on her part. (However, we must keep in mind that both of these disorders may have other origins aside from childhood sexual abuse.)

Only two out of the seventeen patients presented in this book came to treatment because of child abuse. The other fifteen knew they had been abused when they entered treatment, but it was not their presenting problem. Instead, they sought treatment for behavioral or emotional issues related to sexual abuse, but not for the abuse itself, which they disclosed later on. The question that comes to mind is, *Why didn't they come to treatment for the sexual abuse they experienced in childhood?*

The most obvious answer is shame, often coupled with fear of retribution from the perpetrator for telling. Abuse victims expect— and many do in fact experience—disbelief, and/or rejection from their family and others. But there are other reasons.

People who know the patient (including those influencing the girl or woman to get therapy) may miss the connection between the childhood abuse and the self-destructive, socially maladaptive behaviors that follow, including low self-esteem and self-hatred. The depth of these negative feelings is greatly underestimated or misunderstood by the general public. No one approves of hurting children; when the media (newspapers, radio, and television) report or show incidents of children being sexually abused or raped, our reaction is outrage at the perpetrators for committing such a horrendous act against a child. But we generally fail to appreciate the long-term effects of abuse—how this kind of experience changes the child's personality, damaging it possibly for the rest of her life. Abuse—whether one incident or many—is not a momentary scare to be gradually forgotten. Because of this confusion in society at large, most of the patients discussed here also failed to connect their terrible memories with the problems that brought them to therapy.

Of the cases discussed here, five came in presenting anorexia, five were cutting themselves, four were bulimic, and only two were seeking treatment for abuse. I have treated or am treating a total of twenty-seven patients in long-term individual psychotherapy whom I know had experienced childhood sexual abuse. The actual number may be larger, but in the first years of practice I was not looking for this information, which is often not volunteered by patient or family. The proportions of these particular accompanying disorders—cutting, anorexia, bulimia—are typical of all the patients I have seen.

But to fully understand the damage done by child sexual abuse, one must consider both behavioral and emotional consequences. Shame, a feeling of debasement, low self-esteem, and self-loathing can give rise to any of the disorders and symptoms listed below (most of which will be discussed in depth in Chapter 2):

- Aggressively seductive or fearful of others

- Avoids romantic and sexual encounters

- Feels guilt over sexual arousal

- Self-mutilates by cutting or burning her skin

- Anorexia nervosa

- Bulimia nervosa

- Obsessive-compulsive disorder (OCD)

- Early alcoholism and addictions to other substances

- Sleeplessness

- Recurring nightmares involving being pursued by unknown predators

- Genital pain, involuntary contractions and spasms

- Pain when touched nonsexually by others

- Pain when touched sexually by others

- Mood and anxiety disorders

Each disorder or cluster of symptoms represents a personality type, which varies depending on the nature of the child's relationship to the perpetrator and the frequency of the abuse. The closer and more powerful the relationship the perpetrator has with the victim, the more damage she has to contend with. This is compounded by the child's fear that she has no one to turn to for protection. Because of this emotional isolation, she experiences an intensified and negative relationship with her body. To some degree this explains the self-destructive nature of these self-harming disorders. Stuck with these intense feelings of shame and anger, she takes them out on herself.

Shame is of special interest as we discuss the damage and disorders caused by childhood sexual abuse. Because it is at the core of how the survivor relates to herself and society, shame affects all subsequent relationships on both a conscious and an unconscious level. This includes the relationship with the therapist; shame slows down psychotherapy by restricting the patient's ability to confront issues for which she blames herself.

The victim inherits the "shame," disgrace, and guilt the perpetrator would experience if he were caught. Until then, these feelings stay with her unless she confronts him in therapy. The therapist's responsibility is to free her of these feelings so that, even if it isn't possible to confront the perpetrator and elicit a confession and apology from him, she can be persuaded by other means—logic, anecdotes, and pertinent moral references—to revise her sense of self-blame.

2

How Children Survive
Sexual Abuse

Children who experience the trauma of sexual abuse during childhood develop various adjustments to cope with events they cannot understand and feelings they cannot express verbally. When someone experiences physical and/or emotional trauma with no way to emotionally process it, he or she usually develops *post-traumatic stress disorder (PTSD)*. Symptoms of PTSD include some combination of depression, anxiety, recurring nightmares, and flashbacks. Trauma first experienced at any age can produce PTSD, though in childhood it is especially challenging since the child has fewer resources and her mind is still developing. When children have PTSD as a result of childhood sexual abuse, they evolve various defenses, adaptations that help them cope with the stress. These adjustments do not eliminate fears of the original traumatic events or entirely prevent flashbacks or dissociation. Compounding the child's suffering is that dissociation and flash-backs may be triggered by random thought processes—triggered by situations, events, or statements by others that to a "normal" person (in this case, one who has not experienced the particular trauma the child in question has experienced) would seem harmless.

We don't yet understand why PTSD creates the particular adaptations that it does in each person. But we do know that when the trauma is sexual and occurs during childhood, it will, in stages, strongly affect the development of the personality and character of the traumatized girl. Typically, years pass before a victim of child sexual abuse begins psychotherapy, during which time unhealthy defenses and adaptations have developed to help her cope and to enable her to function. These defenses, which we itemized in Chapter 1, vary widely.

A therapist can examine the patient's defenses (adaptations) for their various elements, in order to see how their convergence might explain why she has become the person she is. The process of interpreting her adaptations for her makes her less of a puzzle to herself. In this chapter, we discuss in more detail the defenses itemized in Chapter 1 to see what elements frequently comprise each defense.

SOCIAL AND SEXUAL DEFENSES

Girls who have been or are being abused between the ages of one and twelve may adapt a shy, passive social posture, especially with other girls, and avoid boys whenever possible. This adaptation is not surprising; most of us would find it logical for a victim of any kind of attack to use avoidance as his or her primary social defense. But while some shyness and passivity are tolerated or even expected of girls (depending on the particular community in which the girl lives), having a lot of these two traits is judged by others to be bad. Of course, if we knew the cause of a survivor's shyness, we would feel more compassion for her and less disapproval.

If a woman or adolescent girl fears she's incapable of controlling or limiting unwanted sexual advances, she may rationalize to herself that she can "take it" (being assaulted), in the sense of tolerating it without fear, denying both the pain and the embarrassment. She may adopt an extremely passive posture, sometimes to the point of going limp while being groped, fondled, or penetrated. It is often at these times she will dissociate, becoming oblivious to what is happening to her. This response is usually learned in childhood.

A victim who was abused by an older boy or man when she was a preteen may respond quite differently once she reaches early adolescence. She may become flirtatious and seductive in her manner, wearing provocative, revealing clothing and using body language to emphasize her sexuality. She may take this stance further, becoming sexually active and promiscuous. She may even put up with social disapproval to act this way, because these behaviors are in themselves reassuring to her: provoking sexual interest allows the abuse victim to feel she is in command of sexual activity instead of being victimized by it. Some girls are so inured to abuse that they don't notice society's reaction to this seductive, provocative behavior.

These defensive behaviors are usually compulsive. They create reassurances and feelings of protection for the adolescent or adult who was sexually abused as a child. The need for defenses during sex itself (such as dissociation) remains until the survivor has worked them out in psychotherapy.

Avoiding all sexual contact Some children become sexually aroused while being abused, despite their fears and even their pain. As they grow in adulthood, they experience the sensations of arousal, even when alone, as unacceptable. Instead, the sensation of arousal is usually converted into anxiety, which serves at least two purposes. It reduces feelings of guilt at being "an accomplice" during the abuse, which the arousal implied. It also keeps the feelings of helplessness and despair, associated with arousal during those early experiences, from returning in the present; experiencing arousal would itself be equivalent to revictimization. Since sexual arousal was "stolen" from their control during childhood, it becomes unsafe and unacceptable in adulthood. The result is that arousal is repressed.

Changing sexual orientation   Some women who experienced childhood sexual abuse by men never feel comfortable in intimate relationships with male partners. They may not even be attracted to men or aroused by them. But instead of blocking all sexual feelings, such survivors may transfer them to women, whom they see as safer and kinder, and develop a lesbian sexual orientation. This focus on relationships with women, however, doesn't necessarily solve the survivor's difficulties with sex.

A common theme with some lesbian couples I have treated is the desire of each woman to initiate pleasure for her partner but not be the recipient, because receiving pleasure is too reminiscent of being the passive, involuntary victim of her childhood abuser. When she does allow herself to be the recipient, she may block out feelings of arousal and replace them with feelings of anxiety and guilt. Experiencing her partner's arousal may be the only way she can permit herself to experience her own. But this "solution" to pleasure can bring another problem: as the initiating partner, she now unconsciously identifies with her abuser, whom she remembers as being aroused when he initiated sexually aggressive behavior toward her. Identifying with the abuser, a powerful yet negative role model, may limit the full potential of the romantic love she wishes to achieve.

Women who are generally happy and comfortable in lesbian relationships may still seek therapy to increase their sexual fulfillment and reduce the damage done by abuse. Therapy can help free them of anxiety, guilt, and other negative feelings. Couples work can enhance their capacity for intimacy. Communication about their feelings and histories can improve the trust and closeness they both need. Therapy can also suggest techniques that may be useful. For example, when both partners have the same needs and anxieties, they may find it helpful to keep their eyes on each other during sex to avoid being transported back to "then" and help them stay in the "now." The better they get to know each other, the deeper their relationship can become, increasing their chances of equally pleasing each other.

SELF-MUTILATION

The most common psychological behavioral disorder stemming from childhood sexual abuse is self-mutilation. It can involve cutting the skin with a knife, a razor blade, a pair of scissors, or any sharp or semisharp cutting instrument from bottle caps to broken glass. It may also include burning the skin with cigarettes, matches, lighters, or even chemicals such as lye or acid. Bruising by banging one's limbs on a hard surface is another frequently employed method of self-harming. The significance of the method is that each self-mutilator has chosen a kind of pain and a form of self-damage that *she* can control. She is no longer at the mercy of someone else.

If the response or impulse to self-harm becomes habitual, it can become an addiction. Episodes of self-mutilation may grow more extreme as the cutter tries to prove she is able to put up with more pain and hypothetically (and unconsciously) to better cope with sexual abuse. The behavior escalates in the same way that other addictive behaviors such as drinking, gambling, and binge eating worsen and intensify.

Delicate cutters   Most self-mutilators are cutters. Of these, the majority are what we call *delicate cutters*; they make small (usually three-quarters of an inch to an inch and a half long), shallow cuts that require no stitches. Part of the reason for cutting "delicately" is that they can keep this activity a secret since they don't need to involve medical care.

Acts of cutting are ritualized, each episode lasting five to ten minutes. The ritual involves finding a private place, usually a bathroom; making one or more cuts on the nondominant arm, either leg, or the stomach; watching the cut bleed for five minutes; then washing and bandaging it.

The cutter's experience is twofold. First, the pain from the cutting is reframed into an experience of intensity, which absorbs her current feelings of anger or helplessness and distracts her from painful, often overwhelmingly negative thoughts or feelings. Her self-harm creates a different focus, preventing her from feeling mentally chaotic. Second, the cutter interprets cutting as a way of redressing her grievance, and watching the cut bleed as an acknowledgment of that grievance. In other words, she has substituted her own body for the person of the abuser. Once these needs are momentarily met, she ends the ritual.

Gross cutters   Abuse survivors who endanger themselves by cutting deeper than the two layers of skin are called *gross cutters*. They may cut large veins, arteries, or nerves and lose a dangerous amount of blood. The experiences of the gross cutter may be the same as those of the delicate cutter but more intense. Or she may be cutting during an episode of *dissociation* where she feels detached from time and place, and from her body. The cutter who dissociates is the most endangered since she is not being consciously deliberate and careful while cutting, but rather is mentally unaware and physically numb. She cuts chaotically and recklessly. Gross cutters in general are more likely to have been abused as children, although many delicate cutters may have been as well.

EATING DISORDERS

Anorexia nervosa and bulimia nervosa   Self-starvation by restricting one's food intake, self-induced vomiting, burning calories through laxative abuse or excessive exertion with no goal weight in mind, and the compulsive need to continue these behaviors until other people, or death, intervene—this is anorexia nervosa combined with bulimia. Those who are predisposed to developing these two eating disorders, separately or together, have problems relating to emotional trust, dependency, attachment, and self-esteem. They suffer feelings of inferiority and have conflicts relating to identity and femininity. (Over 90 percent are females.)

The individual who develops anorexia becomes mired in dozens of rigid rules that she creates for herself; these absorb her attention and determine her emotional state. When she follows her rules regarding food and exercise, she feels adequate and balanced but only until the next food-related decision arises. She can also be negatively affected when other people comment on her appearance. This self-imposed mental and emotional preoccupation takes the place of unsolvable emotional problems both past and present. The only relief for her anxiety about these is to obsess over her own weight-loss behavior and the real or imagined slimming or weight loss by others. It is understandable that this self-contained system is preferable to living with unsolvable problems relating to the painful issues mentioned above (dependency, self-esteem, and femininity, among others).

A girl who has been sexually abused sees the goal of pleasing others in order to fend off future attacks as being utterly hopeless. To her it seems better to select a different danger to manage (gaining weight), which to her offers realistic means of prevention (by restricting the intake and hastening the outtake). This is an especially inviting option to anxious and fearful individuals who cannot rely on or develop relationships with others for consolation, reassurance, and protection from their fears and insecurities. Sexual abuse and rape are the extremes in a spectrum of experiences that provoke these feelings. Like the self-mutilator, the anorexic has chosen a solution that is fundamentally self-harming.

Before we continue, a few comments about bulimia are appropriate. As is generally known by now, *bulimia nervosa* consists of overeating or binge eating, followed by some form of purging, most often vomiting. Bulimia nervosa can develop at virtually any age and in either gender. Perhaps because the societal pressure to be thin is still greater for girls and women, the preponderance of cases continues to be diagnosed in females. Bulimia is not necessarily symptomatic of sexual abuse, or indeed any type of abuse, but like the other disorders described here, it may occur as a means of relieving oneself of painful feelings caused by abuse. Briefly, bulimia is an ideal emotional fit for repressed anger in the behavioral cycle begins with pushing feelings down with food and then purging those feelings along with the purged food. (For a more comprehensive examination of bulimia nervosa, see my book *Treating and Overcoming Anorexia*.)

Compulsive overeating   *Compulsive overeating* begins as stress-motivated behavior; it involves eating beyond hunger or necessity, becoming addictive and often leading to overweight or obesity. The act of compulsive overeating, more rapid than normal eating, induces a trancelike state. In the abused person this state serves to block memories and feelings associated with the abuse.

If she sees herself as less attractive due to weight gain, she may also feel safe from further abuse. Alternatively, enhanced emotional safety may result from feeling larger and thus more powerful. Both of these unconscious feelings can override the conscious desire to lose weight, making the compulsive overeating very difficult to give up.

OBSESSIVE-COMPULSIVE DISORDER (OCD)

Obsessive-compulsive disorder (OCD) is characterized by irrational thoughts and fears that intrude on the mind; they are unwanted, but an effort to avoid them only worsens the sufferer's anxiety. In an attempt to allay the anxiety, compulsions to perform repetitive rituals spring up and multiply, since performing them provides only temporary relief. While OCD is a discrete disorder, it can be a feature of a collection of disorders found in survivors of childhood sexual abuse.

Often those suffering with anorexia nervosa appear to have OCD. Because of the repetition of behavior patterns involved in anorexia the rituals may indeed develop an independent energy of their own. This begins with the rigidity of the anorexic's patterns of weight loss behavior and progresses until the rigidity becomes compulsive and superstitious. Departure from the pattern feels too dangerous, for in her mind the anorexic fears that not adhering strictly to her regimens might result in weight gain. The repetition-compulsion proliferates, requiring more and more energy to emotionally provide security from weight gain. The same type of proliferation is seen in someone with true OCD, say the compulsive hand washer, who imagines more and more potential contaminants until she is washing more than one hundred times a day.

However, the anorexic seldom departs from focusing on the (unrealistic) dangers of gaining weight. The compulsive behaviors of the anorexic are all-consuming. In an extreme instance, one woman always held her breath when walking past bakeries for fear of inhaling calories. In some ways these obsessions serve as a refuge from her real fears. When the conscious mind is crowded with thoughts and fears centered on food and weight, there is no room to think about other topics or to feel other fears, such as those connected with sexual abuse.

Self-mutilation also resembles OCD, in that when an abuse victim discovers that physical pain relieves painful thoughts and feelings, her impulses to injure herself take on the same compulsive nature. In girls and women who start cutting in this way, the frequency of the behavior usually increases until it becomes an addiction. Obsessive thoughts about when and where to self-harm can intrude and interfere with normal functioning.

ALCOHOLISM AND DRUG ADDICTION

While anorexia and bulimia may appeal to those who maintain their inner equilibrium using combative self-deprivation and discomfort, alcoholism appeals to those who wish to cope by numbing themselves mentally and emotionally. Feeling overwhelmed by memories and helpless to avoid the feeling that abuse will always be waiting around the corner ("the forever factor") the individual who does not dissociate may choose the emotional anesthesia of alcoholism. Under the influence of alcohol, she also will not be aware of future sexual abuse. Thus alcohol becomes both an anesthetic against memories of past abuse and a vaccine against future pain.

Much of the same can be said about the use of street drugs, particularly cocaine and marijuana. An Australian study of 180 women suggests that "drugs might be used to bolster confidence against anxiety" about further sexual attacks.[3] As with alcohol there is a broad spectrum of reasons why individuals resort to street drugs. Those who start as recreational users and become addicts, as opposed to those who never go beyond occasional use, suffer from more than they can cope with when they are "straight." Genetic factors and family role models can sway the balance in the direction of addiction as well.

Of course, alcoholism and drug addiction by themselves are not indicators of childhood sexual abuse. But these dependencies offer a clue. A 1994 study focusing on the impacts of childhood sexual abuse estimated that, among crisis-center clients, those women who had been sexually abused as children had twice the incidences of alcoholism as the female clients who had not been abused.[4] In addition, the same Australian study mentioned earlier reports *an earlier age* of first intoxication with alcohol or drugs for women who have been sexually abused than for those who have not. So what to look for in a patient, if childhood sexual abuse is suspected, is the early onset of alcohol and/or drug abuse—around ages twelve to fourteen—combined with some of the disorders mentioned earlier.

Blurring this issue to some degree is the precocious involvement of some early adolescents with alcohol, a behavior that can occur in vastly different social circumstances, from urban to suburban, from private schools to economically depressed farming areas. But despite the current "normalcy" of younger drinking ages, true alcoholism in early teens should be noted as a sign of possible childhood sexual abuse.

MOOD AND ANXIETY DISORDERS

Depression and anxiety underlie all of the behavioral disorders discussed earlier. However, many survivors of childhood sexual abuse do not show signs of their victimization through the dramatic symptoms of these disorders. They may appear simply to be shy, quiet, unconfident, low-key children and adolescents. Other survivors adopt postures at the opposite extreme, becoming boisterous, exhibitionistic, promiscuous, angry, flirtatious, and drastically precocious sexually. They may be diagnosed as having *oppositional-defiant disorder, bipolar disorder, borderline personality disorder, suicidal ideation, social phobias,* or one of many other diagnoses. There is no way to tell how many of these diagnoses had their origins in sexual abuse. We often find out ten to twenty years later, when these people enter therapy as older adolescents or adults. Shame may keep them from revealing the abuse for many years or even for the rest of their lives.

FREQUENCY OF CHILDHOOD SEXUAL ABUSE

How frequent *is* the sexual abuse of children? These kinds of assaults may affect as many as 10 percent of children or more, but we are years away from being able to assess the true percentage affected and the damage done to them. The National Crime Victims Research and Treatment Center reports that only 16 percent of adolescent and adult rapes are brought to light.[5] The reports of childhood, toddler, and even infant sexual assault are of course much lower; estimates of the true number will get revised considerably upward when we learn better diagnostic techniques.

The longer the time between when the episodes of abuse stopped (if they have) and when the child tells of the abuse *as abuse*, the greater the damage that has been done to her personality. We have discussed some of the ways childhood sexual abuse affects the victim. Now in Part Two we look at the individual stories of seventeen different women and their courageous efforts to reclaim their futures. We will see how the common thread of abuse connects their lives, and at the same time how distinct each person's story is from the others. Later in the book we will draw on these case histories for the purpose of recognizing different types of abuse, manifestations of trauma, and approaches to therapy.

PART TWO

■

CASE HISTORIES: UNDERSTANDING THROUGH EXAMPLE

3

June:
The Evil Magnet

June's case and treatment history reveal many aspects of childhood sexual abuse: the child's early experience of powerlessness, her attempts to be heard and believed, her self-blame and shame, and when therapy is successful, her ultimate recovery.

June entered the office timidly. She was a shy, attractive twenty-seven-year-old blonde who kept her hair in a nearly boyish bob parted to one side. She stood about five foot seven but despite her height had a slight frame. She had large, blue, wide-set eyes that gave her an expression of both fear and surprise. She seemed nervous about whether to sit on the chair or the couch. While she stood, frozen in indecision, I reminded her in a playful manner, "I get the swivel chair—you can sit anywhere else." She chose the center of the couch behind the small table that contained a box of tissues. She apologetically explained, "I may not look it but I have anorexia. I have gained weight, about fifteen pounds since my low of ninety." I asked her if she had other problems in addition to her anorexia. She looked puzzled. I asked her if she had had problems with depression, anxiety, fears, insomnia, or any other behavior that could be harmful to her.

"Well, I guess I get anxious and depressed, but I don't really know why."

Her manner of speech was both tentative and timid; she talked about her obsession with food and described what seemed like a mild but persistent case of anorexia. We agreed to make a second appointment.

At her second appointment she sat down, then seemed to steel herself for what she had to say. "I believe that you will get bored with me, dislike me, sexually abuse me, and eventually throw me out of therapy."

"Why would I?"

"Because that's what happens to me in life."

"Did you come here hoping for that to happen, or do you hope it doesn't?"

Having spent her energy, she rested her chin on the heel of her right hand. Her elbow was supported by her thigh, the weight of her head causing her to hunch over as she stared at the floor.

"No, I guess I hope it doesn't. But I am used to it happening—especially with men."

"What do you mean by your statement, 'That's what happens to me in life'?"

"I mean, that's how people—men—treat me."

"Is that because you let them, or is it bad luck in your choice of men, or do you choose men who will treat you that way?"

June stared straight ahead for a while. "No, I don't think that it's bad luck. I just can't decide how I would know if a man would behave like that when I meet him. You know they're all nice at the beginning, but after a while they change—they become abusive."

"Do they change because their disguises slip away and that's who they really are? If that's the case we still have to wonder why so many men you choose do turn out that way."

"Do you think I have antennae? Do you think I pick up signals from abusive men?"

"Maybe, or it's possible that you find and develop that part of them that will treat you that way."

She was tearful. "Perhaps it's a combination of both."

"Why might you choose or cause that to happen?"

"I think I'm just used to it." She continued to cry.

"How did you get used to that kind of relation with men?"

"I had good practice . . . for years."

"So this started in childhood?"

She nodded.

"Who was your teacher?"

"My brother was."

"Tell me about him."

"My brother was strange. He was moody, unpredictable, and didn't have friends. He spent his after school time at home, often waiting for me to come home from school when he would pounce on me, and attack me one way or the other."

"What kind of role did he play in your life?"

"In some ways he was like all bratty, bullying big brothers. In other ways he was very different. Sometimes he would tie me up and hit me. Other times he would confuse me by rewarding me for getting good grades in school by buying me toys. My parents never noticed my grades, which were always good. One day he asked me to pull down my underpants. I told him I didn't want to. He said it would be fun. I was still reluctant and he persisted. When he first touched me I said, 'Hey, what are you doing?' He said, 'Touching you in a place where it will feel good.' Then he kissed me on the cheek then on the mouth—quickly and briefly. It was sort of a combination of affection, approval, and sex. All of this was occurring while he was busy touching me in a place that felt tingly and weird. I didn't know what to do. I let him continue. He asked me, 'Doesn't it feel good?' I was confused. It felt wrong *and* good. I felt very guilty after he finished playing with my body. Then the phone rang. It was my mother. She wanted to make sure everything was okay at home and she said she would be back from work in an hour. My brother reassured her we were fine and hung up. That was the first time it happened. I was five years old. He was fourteen. He got more 'experimental' as time went on and I grew guiltier. It continued for years—until I was twelve. He still beat me up at other times just like the 'romance' and sex never happened."

"Did you ever tell your mother what was happening to you?"

"I tried to, but she just couldn't hear it—she didn't even make eye contact with me. I felt so invisible with her. She seemed worried about my brother, preoccupied with him and his problems."

Perhaps because June's parents had been worried about their peculiar son, they had defended themselves from acknowledging the abuse using denial. When June would complain about his assaulting her, her mother would dismiss June's complaints as not being serious. Protection for June was thus out of the question—no end to the abuse was in sight—so she adjusted to the sexual assaults by "getting used to them," as her mother's denial had encouraged her to do.

After a while she found that often she would become aroused when her brother touched her sexually. Thereafter she viewed herself as a coconspirator. Painful abuse became fused with sexual stimulation, which caused her to experience sex as arousal combined with guilt. She was unable to distinguish between them. She felt that these abusive behaviors, directed at her, and her responses to them would follow her forever.

The primary reason June entered therapy was to seek treatment for the personality problems and emotional harm she was suffering currently as a result of being sexually abused by her brother as a child. She stated initially that she was troubled by anorexic ideas. She was embarrassed to state her real reason at our initial session, although she was able to talk about it soon after. She was ashamed of herself for what she had experienced regarding her activities with her brother. She also felt shame for putting up with her relationships with abusive and sadistic men. She described this in our sessions.

"I just don't become attracted to nice guys. I know they would be good for me, but they just don't excite me or arouse me. I go for the guys who don't treat me well but desire me intensely and want lots of sex. Then, after a while I get disgusted with them and annoyed with myself and I stop seeing them, only to go on to the next creep. I have nothing to do with my brother now. He's weird and selfish and still mean, and my mother still worries about him.

She thinks because I'm a successful businesswoman she doesn't have to worry about me. I married a man who was abusive and my mother doesn't know it, but I'm in the process of divorcing him. I'm angry with both of my parents, even though they're nice people and they're nice to me. There's this giant issue between us, which limits my communication with them to simple niceties. I hate the gap between us, but I can't forgive them."

"Do you want to?"

"They'll never hear me. They never have. My brother pretends it never happened, and if it did . . . so what? He actually said that. I don't know whether it's just my brother and my family, but it really seems that everyone thinks that when you're sexually abused, especially when you're young, it's just a bad, scary experience. But I've never been the same since! This 'fooling around' began when I was five and ended when I was twelve. At that point, when he was twenty, he said we could start to have intercourse. I freaked out— it was like a shock, I guess. That's when I got my nerve up and said, 'No more of this, never again!' "

We spent many sessions during which June talked about the negative feelings she had about herself. She made the connection between devaluing her body by seeing it as fat when it wasn't, and devaluing her vagina as the "evil magnet" that seemed to have caused her brother's behavior.

Her relationship with her soon-to-be-divorced husband was different from those with other men she had been involved with in the past. His courtship behavior had been polite, charming, and romantic. After they were married for a year, he began to withdraw from her sexually and she described him as withholding sex as a weapon when they argued. By the end of the second year they were arguing most of the time. He refused to see a marriage counselor. He had a trust fund, which augmented their income, but when it ran out he quit his job and stopped seeking work. He decided to go to graduate school, and she supported them both while he was in school. During this time their relationship continued to become more distant and, according to June, her husband became more argumentative, refusing to have any sexual contact with her. When she entered therapy, she was in the process of deciding whether or not to leave him. She decided she was being abused in the relationship, neglected romantically and sexually, and exploited financially. She filed for a legal separation after several brief discussions with her husband, during which she agreed to wait until he finished graduate school at the end of that year before they divorced. He had threatened to sue for alimony if she didn't agree to this delay. She decided a court case was too much trouble and expense, so she planned to wait the year out. They divorced as per the agreed-on schedule.

Despite the marital conflict, her anorexia faded. She gained an appropriate amount of weight and decreased her obsession with food. But the issue of being attracted to abusive men remained. I asked her if she was ready to have her family of origin come in for a family therapy session. We would use the session to see if her parents were willing to hear her grievances, which, by being acknowledged, could be redressed to some degree. She looked frightened. "My brother will never come," she responded.

"Why don't you call them and ask them to call me? We won't say specifically what the meeting will cover, just that it's for your benefit."

"You don't know my father. He's involved with religion, and he uses it to protect him from anything he doesn't like to be confronted with. Even his clergyman, who he hangs out with like a buddy, talked to him about his avoidance of emotional expression."

"Everyone worries that having their father come to a family therapy session will be a disaster. It never is. Maybe we should have more faith in him."

June called her parents and they eagerly agreed to attend. Her brother was asked by their mother to attend and refused. He indicated that after the family meeting he might consider seeing me alone. His mother found these terms unacceptable and became angry with him but was unable to sway him. Her parents decided to come alone.

When they arrived for the session, we exchanged friendly greetings. I asked June if she wanted to tell them why she wanted this meeting. She proceeded anxiously to explain the abuse. She paused to blow her nose several times. "I told him that was the end of all this and I would go to the police if he bothered me again. I even put the number of the police department near the phone for him to see. And that was the end of seven years of assaulting me."

There was silence in the room. "We never overlooked any of Judd's problems. Why didn't we notice that June was in trouble?" Her father burst out. He was apparently angry with his wife and sad for his daughter.

June's mother patted her on the shoulder. Then she turned sideways on the couch to give June a full hug. "Why didn't you tell us dear?" her mother said after a few moments.

June responded with a lower, more controlled edge to her voice. "I did tell you . . . several times in different ways, but you didn't seem to understand. I believed he had your approval. What else could I think? That's why when he wanted to fuck me I used the threat of the police. I didn't really think they would help, but I was hoping it would scare him off and it worked. He never bothered me again. But that wasn't the end of my problems. It was the beginning. I have unwittingly, or unconsciously, been attracted to men who treat me the way Judd did. I even married one of those men, but that will end soon. It doesn't make me think very much of myself either. And I live in fear that I might trick myself and find another man like that. So I can't trust myself and I can't trust men. I can hardly trust anyone unless I'm in control of the relationship. That leaves me pretty lonely to think weird thoughts, wondering if I'm crazy or not."

June's parents had no response for her, but they were both in tears.

This family session was just one of many significant steps June made in the course of her recovery. For her it was both liberating and validating to finally disclose to her parents the extent of the damage she had suffered at her brother's hands and the effect he had had on her life, her self-esteem, and her relationships. The session served to close the communication gap that had created an emotional estrangement between them. She had finally succeeded in breaking through their denial, and that gave her validation.

As June's therapy progressed, she moved on to the important work of repairing her ability to relate to men in a healthy way. She needed to look at how her brother's abusive behavior influenced her sexual and romantic responses. In one session June described this influence.

"After I got used to his behavior and realized it might go on forever, I had to accept it. I mean, no child has any concept of growing up and becoming more in control of her life. My problem was that in accepting sexual abuse from my brother, I just saw myself as a person who would have to expect it and accept it from others. It's hard to explain to others or even to myself that I expect abuse. It's what I'm used to and I am ambivalent as to whether I mind it or even like it. I wonder if that makes me a masochist or a whore. Intellectually, I know abuse is wrong for me and I hate it, but once it starts, once a guy begins to touch me I lapse into a different set of feelings. Then I think it's okay and maybe I'll get some pleasure out of it. I guess I have been 'trained' for it by my brother, but he's out of the picture now and I'm an adult. I don't know why I can't outgrow the feelings of obligatory submission even if I don't like the guy as a person. Even if I don't like him, when he starts forcing his way into sexual areas he becomes more acceptable."

"So even if there is pleasurable sex, you end up feeling like there's something wrong with you."

"Definitely—like I'm not normal. For a normal woman I know that this sadistic behavior would make the guy less acceptable. She would become angry, take steps to stop him, tell her friends or even the police. She would shout at him, maybe hit him, or push him away. Not me! I become compliant, aroused, and say to myself 'Why not?' My reaction to his behavior makes me hate myself afterward. It's sort of like the person who would like to quit smoking and lights up another cigarette. I know it's bad for me but I get lost in it and forget everything I believe. But it always gets me later. I feel like I deserve anything bad that happens to me, which makes it that much easier to let the next guy do it. I hope I won't always be like this. I feel like everyone can see this in me—especially men. It seems I attract only sexually aggressive guys or I bring that [behavior] out in them. Do I dress or look like I'm easy . . . or worse, like I want to be a sexual victim?"

"No, I think your style of dress is appropriate. But you have brought up an important topic: the childhood abuse has created a pattern of attracting and accepting abusive men. Instead of feeling ashamed of yourself for being victimized by your older brother, you can now use your adult awareness to change this pattern. You can start making better choices, instead of going on autopilot. You can nurture your real self, a person who deserves caring, not abuse. And we can work on assertiveness."

"I don't know—I'm not sure who that real self is or how to identify her."

"I realize that I've laid out a pretty tall order. We should think of these changes as our long-term goals in therapy. They won't happen overnight."

Several months later June brought up serious doubts about herself that reflected her struggle to identify her real self.

"I try to tell myself that I'm different now. But no one can see that. No one can tell who I am. I used to have anorexia and people said to me, 'You're just seeking attention' or 'You're just foolishly stubborn.' No one ever understood that I was compelled to behave like that. It was too terrifying for me to gain weight. So now people think I'm a slut, or I'm stupid, or I'm a wimp. I don't even know if they're right. Am I any of those things?"

"If by 'a slut' you mean someone who wants to capitalize on her sexuality to attract a man for an ulterior motive, other than her being attracted to him, the answer is no. Remember, 'slut' and 'whore' are both pejorative terms used to condemn women who offend others by their promiscuity or infidelity. Do you find yourself in these descriptions?"

"Maybe you're being too generous with me. I don't show discretion when it comes to men. I don't set limits when it comes to how I'm treated."

"I know it's going to take time for you to feel good about yourself when it comes to men. I'd like you to focus on entitlement. You are entitled to good treatment from men and to attention from nice men who are not sadistic to women."

She smiled, "I'm glad to hear that—maybe I'll start to believe it if you say it often enough."

"Okay then, it's a deal."

Treatment for June lasted seven years. She expressed her fears about therapy and the therapist very early on in treatment. This suggests how intense was her fear that she would allow herself to become yet another man's victim. It was more a sign that she mistrusted herself to attract abuse than that she expected the therapist to promote it. As her self-confidence increased, I encouraged her to see me as an ally in her recovery, rather than a person who had more power than she in our relationship. I encouraged her to meet men, when she was ready, and assured her that we would together look for signs that she was repeating the dynamic of attracting abusive men.

We had many discussions about people's behavior during "the courting period" and how to tell what to look for when a man's extraordinary courting behavior faded and his genuine, long-term behaviors emerged. The red-flag signals I alerted her to included the following:

• Controlling her behavior regarding her friends, dress, makeup, and similar

• Possessiveness and jealousy

• Attempts to isolate her from other people in her life

- Premature planning of a future together

- Temper flareups or hints of physical violence

June, in her late twenties, came to therapy naive about dating, though in her business life she was appropriately mature.

June's case provides an unusually clear account of what it's like for a young girl to be the continual victim of sexual abuse by an older brother. Most victims of childhood sexual abuse do not have the clarity to spell it out for themselves or others. As we will see in following chapters, most survivors are blocked by powerful defenses that keep them from consciously experiencing their emotional conflicts.

Over time June began to express her anger at her brother. She became more assertive and blamed her brother for taking advantage of her. She had finally stopped blaming herself for causing the abuse. Learning to place blame on those who hurt her was an immensely important step in June's therapy, producing positive changes in her self-esteem; in time, her better self-esteem improved her relationships with men, friends, family, and employers. As her therapy progressed, June lost her fearful posture and at times was able to disagree with my therapeutic interpretations. She was outgrowing the way she had responded to her brother and other men who had bullied her.

By the time her therapy came to a close, June had begun a healthy dating relationship. She had also made progress in getting closer to her parents. They had stopped denying their son's unrepentant behavior. Her mother accepted responsibility for failing to protect June and distanced herself from her adult son. June finally felt that her parents appreciated her childhood ordeal.

4

Deirdre:
Wanting Family Support,
Not Revenge

Like June, Deirdre grew up in a family situation in which her older brother Davy abused and assaulted her but with no compensating kindness or praise. Again like June, Deirdre's abuse began when she was five, but her brother was aggressive and not "nice" about it. Wanting his approval, she complied with his demands, even though they caused her pain and a clear feeling of being used and devalued. As a result she developed feelings of low self-esteem, and her feelings of inferiority made her shy and withdrawn. These feelings were confirmed by Davy, who told her she was ugly. He convinced her that their relationship was probably her only option, because no other boy would ever be interested in her. The abuse continued until she was twelve.

Deidre felt so intensely dominated by her brother that she believed everything he said. She dressed as plainly as possible and combed her hair in unflattering ways. She succeeded in making herself completely unattractive. This supported Davy's prediction, as even girls excluded her from their social groups. She felt that she had nothing to say that anybody would want to hear. As a teenager she was, to use an old-fashioned phrase, a wallflower. She did not seek out the friendship of other girls nor did she want to have much to do with boys except as distant, platonic friends. Her mother, noticing this, suggested that perhaps Deirdre "had the calling" and should consider becoming a nun; this religious Irish Catholic family already had several nuns, so being a nun was a lifestyle with positive connotations for them.

At fifteen Deirdre developed anorexia. Initially the family denied the seriousness of the problem. After the first year they began seeking outpatient help, and after four years Deirdre started treatment, at which time I hospitalized her. When she began therapy with me, at twenty, she exhibited the same shy personality described earlier for her social interactions. It was only after a dozen sessions that she began to talk about her brother and his behavior toward her. She did so in the voice of someone assuming the listener was only listening out of politeness. She was so soft-spoken as to be nearly inaudible. Her speech was almost expressionless, as though she felt apologetic for taking up the listener's time. My first task in therapy was to continue to listen intently to what she had to say, consistently and over a long period of time. After three months in the hospital she had reached her goal weight and was discharged. She continued with me on an outpatient basis.

An important challenge facing the psychotherapist is to resist the impulse to overexplain to a patient why she is behaving in a way that diminishes or harms her. There is the (unreasonable) hope that the patient's behavior will change immediately upon entering therapy and that the therapist will be gratified at solving her problem quickly. In cases like Deirdre's, therapists have to behave in a manner that demonstrates to the patient slowly, over time, that relationships can be different from the negative ones she has known in the past. If the therapist maintains interest in what she has to say, she will become more confident, and disclose information and feelings she may never have revealed in the past.

Deirdre needed time to talk about the sexual abuse she had experienced and to overcome the feeling that no one would really care. Only then did she explain how she thought the abuse had affected her: "I, uh, just try to stay away from arguments. I try to stay away from people in general, since I never know when they will make me feel bad."

"Are you afraid that they will harm you like your brother did?"

"No, not exactly. I don't imagine them *doing* anything to me. I just get the same feelings as if they might, so I stay away."

I suggested that we have a family session or at least a session with Davy. She refused the session with her family but agreed to meet with her brother. In this session he, unlike most abusers, offered no denials, only the wish to apologize and do anything he could that would make her life and health better. After introducing himself to me, Davy confessed to his sister that what he did was wrong and that he used her, with his assaults, to calm his fears of not becoming a sexually adequate male. He revealed that for three years, beginning when he was seven, his older brother's friend had sodomized him, telling him, "You're gonna be a girl, you're not a boy," and remarking after each act, "See, that's what happens to girls." By the time Davy was twelve, he felt he had to prove his abuser's predictions wrong, so he started to molest Deirdre, convincing himself that he was "the man" and she was "the girl." When she first heard this story—which was new to her—Deirdre found it difficult to mobilize any anger toward her brother.

Davy then shared another story, about being in the navy and getting propositioned by his petty officer to have sex. At this point in his account his tone changed, as he stridently stated that he threw the man out of a second-story window, for which he was discharged from the navy. Davy then described how he would cruise the town at night, looking for gays to beat up. On learning of this violent behavior, Deirdre began to feel her anger toward him. It was then that she suggested the family meet together.

As the session with Davy began, her brother looked uncomfortable. "Why do we need the whole family here?"

But Deirdre's earlier tone had changed considerably. "I'm sorry to hear that you were abused by Harry [his brother's friend], but you presented it to me as if it justified what you did to me, almost as your excuse, until it didn't feel like an apology anymore. When you tell me how proud you are of throwing your petty officer out of a window and that you like to beat up gays, you don't sound like anybody's victim anymore—just someone who's passing on bad behavior. It's like you have become Harry. And yes, I would like to have the family here." Deirdre had found her anger.

"Well I'm not entirely comfortable meeting with Mom and Dad."

"Then we'll meet without you."

"Hey, I came to apologize and you're treating me as a bad guy."

"You did a lot of bad things to me for years and you want to clear your conscience and be forgiven for all that pain and damage in one meeting?"

"I never heard you talk like this."

"I was always too scared of you. No, I was always scared . . . all the time, period."

"Well, I came here to clear it up."

"So come back again to continue to clear it up."

"I think this has become a losing proposition for me."

"You pride yourself on being a good Catholic. Did you ever hear of penance?" Deirdre was wide-eyed and shouting.

When she finished, her expression changed to disbelief at how she had sounded and what she had said. She became tearful, looking as if she wanted to take it all back. In the face of her tears, her brother lost his antagonistic look and shook his head, looking regretful. "I need to think it over," he said, and left.

Deirdre continued to cry in her subdued way. "I said too much."

"I guess you've been saving that up for a long time."

She looked up at me, turned to blow her nose, took a deep breath and sighed, "Yeah."

Davy did not attend the next family session, but both of Deirdre's parents did. Deirdre began to tell them her story: "There were things that happened between Davy and me a long time ago that were wrong. He used to act like he was my boyfriend. I mean he used to do things that boyfriends do to their girlfriends. I was only five when it started. I didn't think I was old enough to be his girlfriend. I didn't like the things he did, but I was afraid to tell any-one about them. He made me feel so helpless." Tears were flowing down her cheeks. Then she checked herself and changed her tone to one of protest. "But somehow he also made me feel like it was *my* fault, like *I* was doing something wrong, that I was bad. Then he lost interest in doing it, and he lost interest in me. He was sev-enteen and I was twelve when it was over. I felt stupid, ugly, and dirty. I still do."

Deirdre's parents were working people. Her father was a steam-fitter approaching retirement, while her mother kept house and baked part-time for a gourmet takeout shop on the other side of town. They were both high school graduates, religious people who understood exactly what Deirdre was telling them, though she was not explicit about the acts themselves. Her father looked angry, though he subdued his expression as much as he could. "I'm throwin' him out of the family. He can never come to our house again!"

Deirdre was taken aback by her father's tough stance. She said, "Maybe this is something we have to talk about. Maybe we have to get Davy to join these sessions."

"I don't want to see him anymore. What he did was wrong, and he didn't even come here like a man to own up to it."

"He came here last week and sort of owned up to it." Deirdre said ambivalently.

"Yeah, sure, I bet he did, and he probably made a lot of excuses like he always did every time he got into trouble."

That surprised Deirdre. She had never thought of her brother except through the eyes of an intimidated younger sister.

"Is that why you always stayed away from boys and hardly have any girlfriends? I mean, you're a pretty girl, and I never understood that. You always dress plain. I don't want to hurt your feelings, I mean, I don't think you dress bad, but you don't dress up much."

Deirdre was in tears, shocked that her father seemed to have noticed so much about her but never said anything to her about these issues before. "Why didn't you stop him?" she cried out.

"Your mother and I never knew. But I'll stop it now. He's out!"

"It's too late to stop it. It stopped seven years ago!"

Her father looked enraged and seemed to want to reassert his role as leader of the family. "I can't have this go on in my family. It's a sin and an evil. I don't want anything to do with him anymore."

Deirdre, for her part, was still looking for someone in her family who would appreciate what she'd gone through and was still going through. She spoke in a more controlled manner. "This family is not helping me. My brother apologizes then excuses, defends, and even glorifies himself. You," she said, addressing her father, "are more concerned with being the boss of the family, and you," gesturing to her mother, "seem to have nothing to say at all. It's clear to me that no one here is concerned with helping me work through what has happened."

Deirdre's father looked taken aback and hurt. "Honey, I just want to see your brother punished for what he's done to you."

"I don't need him to be punished. I need support; I need understanding, which doesn't seem to exist here. You, Dad, you do your masculine thing. Davy did the same thing with his pathetic apology. My mother, the only female in the family, just sits here."

Her mother, looking dejected, finally addressed her daughter. "Deirdre, I'm sorry this whole thing happened to you."

"Well, at least I'm in the picture here. No, never mind, thanks, Mom." Deirdre, who had been tearful through the entire session, seemed exhausted at this point.

I thought we should continue meeting to see if the family could develop its resources to be helpful to Deirdre. "Why don't we schedule another meeting, and why don't you"—I gestured to her father—"see if you can get your son in here to join us."

"Nah, I'm finished with him. I don't want to be in the same room with him."

It was time to end the session. "I want to thank you for coming in this week. I know this has been difficult for you, and I hope you'll think over my suggestion about Davy."

The parents did not return, and the father notified his son of his banishment from the family. Deirdre was not comfortable with this extreme result of her disclosure and kept in contact with her brother, who offered to pay for her college tuition if she decided to attend. She accepted his offer and over the years seemed to forgive him. Despite his initial attempts at excusing himself, he did take responsibility for damaging his sister. The sincerity of her brother's desire to make amends certainly contributed to her recovery.

In therapy we continued to work on the aftereffects of her brother's sexual abuse of her, including her shyness and negative expectations of other people. She worked to overcome anorexia, which had been her adaptation to the abuse, and she learned to assert herself. As the anorexia diminished, she found that she could express herself and use the voice she had heard for the first time in therapy. The overall goal of Deirdre's treatment was to help her move from being a damaged child who became stuck in the past to a healthy young woman who could thrive in the present. This transformation took three and a half years. She is currently married and has several children.

5

Annie and Gina:
Afraid to Receive Pleasure

Annie, a woman in her thirties, came into therapy with the presenting problem of severe anorexia nervosa: Her five-foot-four body was emaciated, and her eyes, nose, and mouth looked too large for her face, which had shrunk to reveal her bone structure. She had thinning hair, a sallow complexion, and her arms were covered with lanugo, a downy growth of hair that many anorexics grow in order to retain body heat in the absence of lost fat tissue. The growth of lanugo can also be provoked by the absence of estrogen, another consequence of female malnutrition. In addition to anorexia, she quickly added a history of childhood sexual abuse at the hands of her grandfather and stepfather.

The initial goal of therapy was to treat Annie's anorexia, which was close to life-threatening. To this end we established a thera-peutic alliance that addressed both the anorexia and the sexual abuse. As she gained weight, her thinking became clearer and the danger to her heart, kidneys, and liver diminished. This took the first year of treatment. Annie went to live with her aunt, who did a lot of cooking for her. Unlike rebellious, angry anorexics, Annie was grateful for her aunt's help. She cried a lot in our sessions about how she should never have allowed herself to do this much destruction to her body.

As an adult free of those who abused her against her will, Annie prior to therapy had engaged in *consensual abuse*. She would pick men up in bars, take them home, and ask that they penetrate her in various painful ways that she suggested. She was always drunk from the time she met the men until the dangerous acts were completed, after which she would fall asleep. She would wake up in pain the next morning barely remembering what had happened. Often she would not remember at all, thanks to her alcoholic blackouts. The physical damage she suffered was so severe as a result of some of these episodes that she required surgery.

During the course of therapy she realized she was gradually becoming attracted to women and losing her romantic and sexual interest in men. She developed a relationship with Gina, another woman with a long history of sexual abuse, in this case by her father and two brothers. Annie moved in with Gina, and within two months they developed problems in their sexual relationship. Annie asked if Gina could come in to meet me and if the two of them could have couples sessions.

In contrast to Annie, whose manner was mildly androgynous, Gina looked and dressed distinctly like a man. She entered the office after gesturing to me to enter first, saying, "I can't have you walking behind me." Her gait, voice register, and facial gestures were extremely masculine. She swaggered in, spoke in a deep voice with a hint of physical threat, and looked around the room like a detective looking for evidence.

"So we sit on the couch?" she asked in her raspy voice, her annoyed tone aimed at Annie.

Annie didn't answer but sat on the couch, then Gina sat next to her. Annie began, "Gina and I have a sexual problem."

Gina interrupted, looking at me, "Oh, is he going to be in bed with us?"

"In a manner of speaking, yes," I answered.

She narrowed her eyes at me. "You know, I trashed my last shrink's office."

"I guess you were mad at him."

Annie interrupted, "Gina, can I continue?"

"Yeah, yeah."

"You are the first woman I have been with. You don't let me touch you. You have to be the doer, never the receiver. If I wanted that, I could be with a man. The reason I'm with a woman is, among other things, to be physically involved with *her body.*"

Gina was suddenly quiet.

"Does Annie's request make you uncomfortable?" I asked Gina.

"It's not easy for me. Maybe I'll get used to it in time." Gina's tough, defiant attitude showed signs of softening. She looked uncomfortable and embarrassed, struggling to keep her composure.

"Gina, does Annie's complaint have anything to do with you not being comfortable with me walking in behind you?"

Gina looked up at me, startled, and became tearful. "You don't know what they did to me! They did it whenever they wanted to. It was both of my brothers and my father. Oh yeah, they were a great team." She punched the arm of the couch and clenched her jaw. "I can't talk about it any more. I can't stand this!"

Annie was intimidated by Gina's expression of pain. The focus of the session then moved away from Gina, who spent the remaining time looking at the paintings on the walls of the office and trying to recover. Annie tried to take Gina's hand, but she pulled away saying, "Just let me sit here, okay, Annie?"

I continued to meet with them together, spending several sessions focusing on Annie's history. This took the pressure off Gina— and off Annie as well since she had already revealed much of the material in individual sessions. Annie recalled that her first encounter with sexual abuse was with her grandfather when she was three years old. Abuse by him continued sporadically and alternated with abuse by her stepfather, which began two years later, when she was five. Annie also described again the abuse she had invited as an adult by taking strange men home from bars and suggesting "rough sex"—erotic activities that were often harmful and painful to her. One of the bars was a "cop bar," as Annie put it, since its clientele were mostly police officers. She would suggest "creative ways" they could use their nightsticks and always found a few takers. Her anorexia was her first attempt to escape the masochistic activities she had engaged in with men. When she gave these activities up, partially due to internal injuries she had sustained, her anorexia developed. (Sexual masochism involves experiencing sexual arousal through the infliction of pain by one's partner.)

After listening to these stories, Gina became more willing to talk, in nonexplicit terms, about her own experiences with her father and her two brothers, but revealing these was a gradual process.

As the weeks went by Gina dressed and postured less as a caricature of tough maleness. Even the raspy strident quality of her voice changed. During this period she questioned Annie, in a supportive manner, about the information Annie was sharing with her for the first time. Gina sensed that it was becoming her turn to share her well-kept secrets.

At the start of the session in which the focus shifted from Annie to Gina, Gina offered me a candy bar. "Hey Steve, do you like Milky Ways?"

"Sure. Thanks, Gina."

"Maybe there *are* some good guys," she said as she walked over to the couch. I was touched by Gina's new ability to relinquish her guarded posture. She seemed ready to take a big step in couples therapy.

"Gina, nobody wants you to describe what's been done to you in graphic terms," I reassured her. "We don't want to watch, to see what has been done to you. It would be helpful if you could talk about your vulnerability because of these events so that we can begin to distinguish between 'now' and 'then'—between Annie, and your brothers and father. Annie is not a predator. She doesn't want to harm you for her own excitement the way your family did. She wants to please you. That would be exciting for her."

Gina looked thoughtful. "But what if I can never make the distinction you talk about? What if I'm stuck there and can never feel like it's different? What if I always feel raped, humiliated, and tricked, even though it's Annie? That wouldn't be sex for me. That's torture."

Annie took Gina's hand. "If you can't trust me, how can we be together? I know it can't happen overnight, but I have to know you're trying."

Gina looked down at their intertwined hands, nodding wordlessly. During the next few months Gina became more relaxed as she accepted that not everyone was a potential predator, especially not Annie.

Annie and Gina continued to come to therapy as a couple, ultimately deciding to move out of New York City to a small town upstate, where they found a social work agency at which to continue their treatment.

By working together in therapy Gina and Annie had each been able to revise their feelings about trust and relationships. In this case Annie had had a head start with her achievements in individual therapy; she was then able to help her partner move forward. Like most couples, their most important goal was enhanced communication, learning to meet one another's needs through mutual listening. They had difficulty with learning to experience trust and comfort in a physically intimate relationship. Achieving this aspect of closeness is especially challenging for people who have suffered childhood sexual abuse. Gina's deep emotional scars and Annie's extremely self-destructive behavior emphasize the extent and intensity of the damage that victims carry with them into their adult lives.

6

Adrienne:
Sad Little Girl in the Photo

drienne was a twenty-one-year-old high school graduate when she was referred to me for abusing alcohol, marijuana, cough medicine, and a variety of other substances. She had also been cutting herself. Adrienne was an unusually tall (six feet), attractive girl who was living in a blended family with her mother, stepfather, and two sisters. She stated she was suffering from depression and severe insomnia.

The reason she was experimenting with all these substances was her desire to fall asleep and stay asleep throughout the night. Adrienne had recently moved to her own apartment; her family was affluent, so the expense was inconsequential. Adrienne often went out to clubs, where she drank and danced with a number of friends. She had just broken up with her boyfriend and seemed to be trying to compensate for her loneliness.

Though Adrienne did go out a lot and danced with many boys, she was a *serial monogamist*: she always had just one boyfriend at a time. But the young men she became involved with often exploited her, were lazy, lived in her apartment, paid none of the rent or phone bills, and had her do all the food shopping, for which they contributed no money.

After Adrienne and I had met a dozen times, I asked her if she had ever been sexually abused. She stared straight ahead for a minute and said, "Yes I was, often, by my uncle. When I was a little girl, he would take me into the ocean, and while holding me mostly above the water, he would penetrate me with his fingers. When I would protest, he would insist that we were just having fun, playing a game, and that I should be a sport and enjoy the game. He would always say this with a hearty laugh that made me feel like a killjoy. I wanted to tell my mother but I was always hearing that my uncle and his wife—my mother's sister—were having marital difficulties. It seemed that my mother was afraid that they might get divorced. I didn't want to cause trouble between my aunt, who I liked, and my uncle, who I hated. I was also afraid that my mother would be mad at me or not believe me. I guess I thought their marriage was the paramount concern."

The following week Adrienne brought in pictures taken of herself at different ages, both alone and with her family. "Do you see how I was frowning and looking miserable in all of the pictures?" she asked.

"Yes, everybody is smiling but you."

"Don't you think someone should have noticed? But no, nobody ever did. I knew it would go on forever or maybe until I became too big for him to do that. I always hated him and thought about killing him. I dreaded it when my mother would say, 'Let's go for a picnic lunch at the beach,' which was every week in the summer. He would look at me and smile. Finally I did get too big for him to try that. When he asked me to go in the water with him, I just glared at him. I don't even know if he got the message, but he backed off and went in the water by himself."

Adrienne's manner in telling her story was not sad like that of many other abuse survivors; instead, at this point in the therapy, she maintained a steady, angry tone. This would change later on.

After a severe bout of cutting Adrienne was hospitalized to prevent her from further endangering herself. While at the psychiatric hospital she met a young man a few years older than herself. He was remanded to the hospital as an alternative to prison for using large amounts of cocaine. Adrienne developed a crush on him.

After they were both discharged, she kept in contact with him and over her parent's objections decided to pay him a visit. During the course of the evening his behavior changed and he began to assault Adrienne and then raped her. She didn't want to press charges, but I notified the hospital and they put him on the No Admit list. Adrienne indicated that this was not the first abusive boy she had been involved with. When she realized her role in attracting and accepting abusive behavior, her sadness finally emerged.

"I can't believe what my uncle did to me! That bastard! I thought he just molested me, but really it's like he changed my whole personality. I've been drinking and taking drugs to fall asleep . . ." Her angry tirade gave way to weeping.

"Adrienne I know this is hard, but you need to have your feelings—it's that or you wind up taking it out on your body by hurting yourself."

"I know that's true," she sobbed, "but this hurts more than cutting myself."

"I'm thinking of that photo you showed me, the sad little girl who couldn't tell anyone that her uncle was hurting her. She's been trying to deal with that pain for a long time, and it hasn't been working."

"No it hasn't. And I'm tired of hurting myself instead of him and finding other men to treat me like I'm worthless. I always knew he was the bad one, and yet I ended up accepting the abuse."

This was the first step in Adrienne's breakthrough, the first time she realized that she was reliving her past, that her angry demeanor was a coverup for her real pain. After this, her therapy was somewhat of a rocky road for a while. After giving up alcohol and cutting she went through a period of overeating, but eventually she conquered that as well.

An important theme throughout her recovery was her recurrent attraction to aggressive men and drug users. After exploring this tendency she vowed to stay away from any romantic involvements unless the man behaved in a gentle and sensitive manner. We also decided that Adrienne should get to know some of a man's friends, so she could better judge his character.

"I guess I'd better stay away from my uncle's look-alikes."

Adrienne's reaction to her abuse was unusual in that she did not blame herself. On some intuitive level as a child she understood that her uncle was being sneaky and that he was the one at fault. She also realized that pressure was being put on her not tell on him in order to protect her mother's sister. This gave her a perspective or context whereby she was able to feel anger rather than terror. In her teenage years she had acted out with delinquent behavior and, despite her subordination to her boyfriends, held a position of leadership with other girls. She was stylish and flirtatious in an assertive style, until she got in trouble with substances and drifted toward boys who were abusive to her, even in nonromantic relationships. Because she had allowed her feelings of anger to emerge at the time of the assault by her uncle, recovery for her was quicker than for most survivors—about two years.

Adrienne's story is significant because it illustrates the way in which she re-created her childhood abuse by selecting an addict remanded to a psychiatric hospital. Low self-esteem creates this pattern in many abuse survivors. For Adrienne this sexually abusive man was reminiscent of her uncle, in that they were both self-serving and sadistic.

When women heal and regain their self-esteem, they gain the ability to recognize a person or relationship that echoes the early abuse. Then they can put an end to the self-destructive patterns and make better choices.

7

Marjorie:
Uncle Bill in the Barn

Marjorie was originally referred to me for treatment of anorexia nervosa. She was nineteen years old and a college freshman with a three-year history of the disorder. Her comments didn't express the usual body distortion talk that typically comes with anorexia. That is, she didn't complain about imaginary fatness or claim that she ate like a pig. She did talk about the need to be thin, but it was to feel safe, not socially adequate. "It's important to make sure I don't gain weight and look normal. It's safer." She stated this frequently, including comments about not eating "dangerously," referring to eating too much. When I asked her what made normal eating and appearance dangerous, she explained, "If you are shapely, boys like to bother you, to touch you."

She described a date in which the boy had put his arm around her as he drove the car and slowly but obviously lowered it down from her shoulder until his hand was on her right breast. He fondled her for a while until the car came to a stop at a red light. He turned to kiss her, only to discover she was silently crying, with tears streaming down her face. He took his hand away and said, "I thought you'd like that. Other girls do. What's the matter?"

She tried to stop crying and said, "Could you just take me home please?" That ended the date.

She withdrew from dating boys for months after that and continued to lose weight. Since her appearance made her quite unattractive, she received very few requests for dates.

She explained, "I can't say no to anyone about anything. I can't say 'stop' or 'don't' either. I never could. The only thing I can do is try to make it not happen in the first place. If I'm thin enough they won't ask me out. If they ask me out anyway, maybe they won't want to touch me because there's nothing to touch."

"Why do you think it's difficult for you to state how you don't want to be treated?"

"I don't know. I just never could."

"Do you remember the first time you were treated by someone in an objectionable way?"

Marjorie became silent, then tearful. She sat there for a while crying and then began. "When I was little, I don't remember how young, my mother's brother, my uncle, would take me out to our barn—we lived in the country then—and he would touch me there," she explained, pointing to her crotch. It seemed he was having fun. He was doing all sorts of things to me. It could last a half hour. I didn't say anything and that was okay with him. I didn't move. Sometimes he would pinch me there just to make me squirm. I think he liked it when I squirmed or said 'ouch.' He told me, with a mean expression on his face, 'You'd better not tell anybody about this or they'll think you're a bad girl.' This went on for over a year, and then I asked my mother what it means when a grown man touches a little girl. She dismissed it and said, 'When I was a young girl, we all put up with some of that. We just learned to ignore it. Men are pigs.' I had nobody to turn to for protection. Three years later I asked my sister—I think I was ten by then—if Uncle Bill had ever done that to her. She looked surprised and said, 'Yeah, but nobody cares.' He stopped when I got my first period. I told him I was going to tell on him if he didn't stop. He stopped. I didn't think I could threaten him. I tried to tell my mother and it didn't work. Maybe he was right. If I complained about him, I might be thought of as a bad girl or a liar. Whenever he visited he'd grab me and sit me on his lap. He'd hold me there and bounce me on his lap. Something about it felt disgusting. So I learned to be passive, go limp at the same time as I was tense. That's what I do now—I can't seem to change that. Anyway, I learned to hide when I knew he was coming over with my aunt. I either left the house or if I had no place to go, I could spend hours hiding under my bed. I could hear him asking for me, but my mother would dismiss his request just as quickly as she dismissed my questions about girls being molested. I think she knew something, but she never talked to me about it. After all, he was her older brother."

Marjorie and I decided to have a session with her older sister, who was then twenty-four. She corroborated Marjorie's experience and we discussed the possibility of having a family session. Neither sister was ready to include their uncle in a confrontation, nor did we ask their mother to attend, feeling she was burdened with her own terminally ill mother. We decided to start by having a session with their father.

The sisters' father, Eddie Franks, was a tall, sturdy, man. He had done physical work his whole life and ran a furniture business. He sat down in my office looking mystified. Trying his hand at humor, he asked, "Am I in trouble?"

"No, Mr. Franks, you're not in trouble." I reassured him. "But your daughters want to tell you about experiences they have had which were not good for them." He looked relieved and curiously intense at the same time. Each girl told about her episodes with Uncle Bill. The more they talked the redder his face became, the angrier he looked. When they stopped he asked them, "Why didn't you tell us this was going on?" The girls looked at each other; they didn't want to betray their mother's insensitivity to their disclosures.

"We didn't think that anyone would believe us," said the older sister. "Uncle Bill threatened us never to tell or we would get into serious trouble. I thought he would kill me."

"I'd like to kill him!" was the father's first response.

We all sat in silence waiting for a second response.

"The barn, huh, this all happened in the barn? He and I will have to have a talk in the barn. You know, he's a social worker with young children. God knows what he does to them or how many others he's harmed in addition to my girls."

At her next session Marjorie told me what happened. "Last Sunday Uncle Bill and his wife came for a visit. My father looked at us, and turned to Uncle Bill and said 'Bill, let's take a walk. There's something we need to discuss.' We saw Uncle Bill looking uncomfortable. This was not my dad's style and he seemed on edge. Perhaps Uncle Bill's guilt made him nervous. We were excited. Maybe my dad would make him pay for what we went through. We watched them go into the barn. I heard my uncle say, 'Now don't tell me you bought a horse, Eddie.' Later my father relayed the following conversation to my sister and me:

"Bill, both of my girls sat me down in a therapist's office and told me about all the sexual things you did to them when they were younger. I believe them. I believe you're a sick bastard who shouldn't be around children. I'm calling your supervisor at the Bureau of Child Welfare and telling him or her about this. Furthermore, you're going to apologize to my girls for what you've done to them, and don't try to make excuses or blame it on them or I will go beyond the law with you. You see that axe handle over there? No court will convict me, you miserable child molester . . ."

I saw your uncle start to sweat when I stood right next to him for emphasis. "Now I am going to ask the girls to come in here and you *will* apologize in front of me. Do I make myself clear?"

"But Eddie, I'll lose my job again—I'll never be allowed to work in social work. I'll be labeled under Megan's Law! Our lives will be ruined."

"How much of my girls' lives have you ruined? How many other lives have you ruined?" Then I paused. "Okay, if you apologize and you resign from your job and never work with kids again, I'll let it go at that."

"And Uncle Bill did what my father told him to do. He apologized to Angela and me that afternoon. I was surprised because, instead of feeling satisfied, I felt so angry I thought I wanted to kill him. I mean, I would never kill anybody but that's how angry I felt toward my rotten uncle. I was surprised because I never get angry at anyone."

"Maybe now you will be able to get angry at people who hurt you instead of turning it against yourself."

Marjorie looked startled at the suggestion that she might have to make such a change.

"Well maybe not so fast and not so complete, but it could be a beginning . . ."

"Yeah, I guess it could be," she nodded.

Marjorie and I set up tasks and exercises to develop assertiveness, and confrontation and protest with others (see Chapter 26). During the course of therapy Marjorie married and had a baby girl. This was complicated by a fear that she wasn't ready for motherhood. During her first trimester of pregnancy Marjorie began to lose weight. Her obstetrician told her that she was two centimeters dilated and she could lose the baby. We had to work quickly on this.

I began to feel as if we were thrown back to the time when Marjorie was actively anorexic because we were again struggling with issues from her earlier therapy. "You are looking thinner each week Marjorie."

"Um, yeah I think I lost a little weight."

"I think you're trying to starve that pregnancy to cause a miscarriage."

Marjorie became tearful and nodded. "I wanted to do this in six months—not yet."

"You have committed yourself to this pregnancy for ten weeks now. Do you want to lose the baby?"

"I don't know. I'm scared."

"We spent a lot of time discussing your getting pregnant. You seemed decided that you wanted a baby."

"I think I do." She continued crying.

"Marjorie, when a woman takes the best possible care of herself during her pregnancy and the baby is imperfect she feels guilty. If you produce a damaged baby after starving nearly to the point of a miscarriage, you will never forgive yourself whether I say this or not. You have to gain back the necessary weight quickly, and we have to find other ways for you to deal with your self-doubts about becoming a mother. I'll help you during your pregnancy and afterwards for as long as it takes."

She came to her sessions and worked on her eating until several days before she gave birth. When her baby daughter was ten days old, Marjorie brought her to our next session. Pointing to the small carriage containing the tiny sleeping infant, she began, "She is going to like my husband better than me. She will find him smarter, more interesting, and more fun than me. She'll want to be with him more than with me." Marjorie looked sad and resigned.

I was struck by the incongruity of the complex series of attitudes Marjorie was predicting for her daughter, in contrast to the reality of this newborn baby, for the moment asleep and oblivious to the world. "That's quite a program you're imposing on that adorable little 'blank slate' sleeping over there."

"I just don't feel that I can be very valuable to her. I've never felt I could be valuable to anyone. I don't even know if it's just me or all girls and women . . . I do feel like it's me though."

"But it's different for men?"

"It must be. Look what happened to my sister and me. According to my mother—who was born in the old country—girls just have to put up with anything men want to do to us. My father scared my uncle Bill, but my sister and I still needed a *man* to take care of it. I guess, compared to men, women aren't so important."

"Wow! That's a sweeping indictment about women, isn't it? First of all, you and your sister deserved to have your father step in and set things right with your uncle; it was long overdue. As for importance, you're talking about size, age, and physical strength, aren't you? When you were little, you were overpowered by a man who was bigger and stronger than you were. Even in your adulthood this could still happen. But should we allow comparative physical strength to determine the *value* of one gender over another? How do you want your daughter to feel about *herself*? Should she perpetuate the way you are feeling about yourself now?"

"No, I don't want that for her."

"Then we can't have that for you either. She will copy what she sees in your eyes."

"So I have to save me to save her from becoming me?"

"Yes, I believe so."

Marjorie worked on self-esteem for quite a while. We discussed the value of femininity and the damage her uncle had done to it. She allowed herself to feel important in her daughter's life. She took her to swimming classes, gymnastic classes, dance classes, taught her to read at three, and spent a lot of time cuddling with her. Her daughter thrived on Marjorie's attention, just as she enjoyed her father's company, playing sports with him, and growing in a healthy, balanced family.

Marjorie's story illustrates two important points related to recovery from childhood sexual abuse. One is the powerful role played by confrontation of, and apology by, the perpetrator. A turning point in Marjorie's treatment occurred when her father confronted her uncle and made him apologize to his daughters. In preparing for this event, Marjorie's family and I had established that the apology specify that her uncle was solely responsible for his behavior, that the abuse was no fault of theirs, and that he regretted damaging and upsetting them. What makes this kind of apology effective is that it weakens the perpetrator in the survivor's eyes and diminishes her fear of the "forever factor" (that men would always abuse her and she would always have to adjust to abuse).

Another reminder occasioned by Marjorie's story is that, when we hear about child sexual molestation, it is important to think about the "stolen tomorrows" which, if the survivor does not recover sufficiently from her abuse, may extend to her children.

8

Lana:
"Easy Money"

Lana came to treatment at the age of eighteen after dropping out of a highly competitive college toward the end of the first term. She gave bulimia as her reason for dropping out.

Lana and her family emigrated from South Korea when she was ten years old. She was an attractive girl who continuously wore a grin on her face that occasionally broke into a smile, though her eyes were unsmiling. She was about five foot ten, slender, with long hair wrapped coquettishly around her neck emphasizing her neck's length. She said that although her mother insisted she enter treatment for the bulimia, there was a second reason her mother wanted her to get therapy.

Lana with no prompting smilingly explained: "I just didn't feel comfortable at college. It was a very conservative New England school and all business. I quickly got the message that everyone was serious about their future as were their parents. There were parties on Thursday nights where everyone drank beer until they either passed out or vomited. Some of the girls threw up out the windows, and it became a contest [to see] how far it went. For a college there wasn't a lot of sex and not too much drugging. I didn't belong there. I felt like a freak, not because I'm Asian but because I'm from New York, which made me suspect—and for good reason. The place was square! This stressed me out and made my bulimia worse. I had developed it in my senior year at high school. I felt so alone and alienated, I thought about suicide. I figured I'd better leave, even though the dean tried to convince me to stay."

She paused just long enough to take a breath. "I got a job last week that pays five hundred dollars a night. More than I could make if I graduated that school. I act . . . well, kind of . . . I mean, in porn movies. I was nervous the first time but now I'm doing it, completely naked, and I don't care. I just don't care about myself in general. I just feel that they can use me because I don't matter— I'm worthless anyway. Yeah, I guess you could say I'm depressed, but the label doesn't help me with the feeling, it doesn't change anything. So my feelings of worthlessness give me the freedom to make five hundred dollars a shoot. I don't know if my family knows. I think they have an idea, but they won't mention it. But I bet my mother sounded real intense about me coming into treatment, maybe more intense than other mothers whose daughters have bulimia?"

"Yes, your mother sounded very frightened and desperate about it."

"My mother often sounds like that. She's had a panic disorder as long as I can remember. I guess that's why I could never go to her with my problems. She's not the kind of person you can lean on; she just falls apart."

"That must have made you feel a little lonely. I'm not surprised you've been scrambling to come up with your own solutions. I've always thought that bulimia is an attempted solution for emotional isolation."

"I never thought of that, but I guess it makes sense." Lana was doing her best to stay casual in this conversation but her voice was shaky and her smile had faded.

"So now you're trying to solve the financial problem by acting in pornographic movies. You know, your mother said they could afford treatment, but if they had to, they would take a loan."

"Yeah, that sounds like my mother—she could sell our house in a panic. And it's a nice house in a cool town in Pennsylvania."

Her face changed expression again, this time giving me a tired, cynical smile. I was reminded that she had taken a three-hour train ride to see me. "I told them I could afford to pay for therapy easily," she went on. "That worried them. I shouldn't have said that. That's probably how they figured out I was up to something shady."

"You are telling me that even though your parents expect to pay for therapy, you want to pay me with money you earn from porn?"

She shrugged her shoulders and cocked her head. "Sure, why not? It's easy money and no strain on them."

"It doesn't seem to be 'easy money.' How's your bulimia . . . how frequent?"

"Three or four times a week."

"What about your self-esteem?"

"I don't care what happens to me. I guess I feel even more worthless having sex in front of a camera, but I want to get used to doing it because it pays so much money."

"Have you taken a good look at your employers?"

"Yeah, some of them are really sleazy and disgusting."

"So that's who you're working for, and of course the people who will see the films."

"I don't like to think about it. I try not to see them when I'm on the set."

"How will you be able to keep it up?"

"One of the other women, a nice person, offered me some coke. I turned it down, but I think that maybe someday, if it's more than I can handle, I'll try it. The manager had mentioned threesomes to me, or maybe lesbian stuff—with a raise. That might push me over the edge and then I'll need the coke."

"You say it so passively, like you're resigned to it."

"Hey remember, I don't care about myself, and with the raise it will be another two hundred a pop."

"Okay, I need to establish an important ground rule. You can't pay me with money you earn from any sexual service occupation. I can't control what you do with this money, but your parents can pay for the therapy. You can't tell me that you have to be a porn actress to pay for therapy since your parents are willing to help you. You've owned up to the destructive side effects it's having on you—lowering your self-esteem, driving you to use cocaine. Who knows how bad it'll get."

"But that's . . ." her voice trailed off to a deflated sigh.

"Your sex film money is no good here. If that was how you had to support yourself it would be different, but you are at the beginning of a behavior which will harm you and you have a choice."

Lana didn't come back for a month. I received a call from a hospital emergency room in Pennsylvania. Lana had told her girlfriend she was going to kill herself, and her girlfriend had called the police. When brought to the hospital Lana gave them my business card and told them she was my patient. When she was discharged two days later, her mother once again called me, without mentioning the hospital episode, and asked if Lana could resume treatment. Lana complied with her mother's wishes and returned to therapy.

At our next session Lana explained that the situation at work was becoming more oppressive: the male filmmaker had begun assaulting her both physically and sexually, so she resorted to using cocaine since it made her less sensitive to her brutal environment; this allowed her to keep earning what was now seven hundred dollars a day. She had become so depressed at the situation she was trying to find acceptable, and at the same time so torn about losing her high income if she left, that she had become despairing and suicidal.

In the following session she told me, "I'm thinking of becoming a lesbian. I've fooled around with one of the women at work, and it's working for me. I'm becoming paranoid and feel like I hate all men, and I'm ready to pick a fight with them in the street, even if nothing has happened. There's another part of me that would like to 'flash' them and walk away, just to tease them—you know, get revenge."

"Maybe you should continue your lesbian experiment to see if it works. You certainly have enough reasons at this point to hate the men you're surrounded by every day you go to work. I'm sure they seem like they represent all men to you now."

"I have more reasons to hate men than you know."

"Do you think that these reasons have something to do with you wanting revenge?"

"Yeah, I do. Maybe one of the reasons I felt drawn to working in the sex business was because of what happed to me when I lived in Seoul, Korea. My cousin, who was ten years older than I . . . let me think . . . I was five and he was fifteen. He used to undress me when we were alone on weekends. He would say it was a game. He even said it was a game they played in America and America saved us from being killed by North Korea, so it must be a good game. The game came down to him taking off one piece of clothing after another, slowly, including my underwear. Then he would make me lie down, pull my legs apart, and penetrate me in both places for a long time. Then when he thought our parents were returning, he put my clothes on as fast as he could. I hated the game, but he made it sound so normal I didn't complain to my parents. I was afraid to and I don't even know why. Maybe I thought they would be mad at me for doing it, or complaining about it, or getting my cousin in trouble, and I was sure he would get even with me for that. So that went on for three years. I once saw him with a girl who looked about eighteen at that time. I guessed he found someone his own age to play the game with."

"Did you feel relieved?"

"This is going to sound crazy, but I felt a little jealous and rejected. I think that was the beginning of my feeling worthless. I wasn't even good enough to be used by my cousin."

"Do you think there's a connection between what your cousin did to you and your becoming involved with performing sex acts publicly?"

"There must be a connection, but it's confusing. This week during a film shoot, a cameraman tried to penetrate my butt. I shot up in the air with shock, got dressed, and walked out of the 'money mill.' I guess it reminded me of my cousin's game.

"When I was between six and seven years old, I did ask other older girls if they ever heard of that game. They laughed at me and said, 'It's not an American game—it's a Korean game.' They said, 'It's part of being a girl growing up in Korea for a lot of us.' So in Korea I would be trapped, but here, I could walk out of the movie business even if it hurt to give up the money. That was the day I thought I would kill myself. I had dropped out of college, didn't know where I belonged, and couldn't earn enough money to support myself."

Her expression was skeptical—a wry smile formed. "No future for me, eh?"

"One person's behavior toward you has affected your life and the way you feel about yourself so severely, it seems like the way you feel today will last forever. We must help you believe that you are still capable of growth that will make living worthwhile."

"And how do we do that?"

"If you're here, you can't be all pessimist. Are you afraid to hope?"

"I'm less hopeful than ever because I have lost all sense of modesty. I didn't really need the coke anymore by the time I quit. I could look at the men on the set and laugh inwardly to myself. If I don't care about being naked, I'm worth more money than I could get paid at any college graduate's job. It makes my self-esteem go up and down at the same time. I don't quite get that part. What's that about?"

"The money makes you feel 'worth more.' But what you're doing for it and whom you're servicing makes you feel worthless. It confirms the problems you had before you started to work at this. After all, you earn a lot of money not because you are skillful or educated, but because you put yourself on exhibition in front of men you would find disgusting and who will masturbate while watching you. Not much prestige in that, is there?"

"Yeah, I guess I always knew that was back there but didn't want to think about it. You see? I'm really worthless now."

"You have been involved in work that makes you feel like that. Will you quit the sex business permanently so we can work toward helping you recover your sense of value?"

"I hope it works."

"You won't be doing this on your own, you know."

"I'm counting on that or I have no chance."

Many young people have not yet become healthy enough or independent enough to leave home to live in a residential college. In Lana's case, issues concerning her mother's panic disorder during her childhood, compounded by her cousin sexually abusing her in childhood, impaired her development of the security and trust from which independence springs. Without a sense of security at home, she was vulnerable to the bulimia she developed at school, along with the strong sense of alienation she experienced among the other students. Adolescents in general have difficulty thriving in college if they leave home without a strong sense of security. They must feel that even over long distances, home and parents are only a phone call away. They can be reassured should they feel anxious about friends, schoolwork, dating, finances, and even minor illnesses. These are the major reasons undergraduates call home and, in severe cases, return home.

Lana's childhood sexual abuse put her at high risk for "breaking down" during her freshman year. Because of her mother's mental illness, Lana had missed out on experiencing *basic trust*, an important building block of healthy development that allows a young person to form an individual identity when he or she goes out into the world. This unresolved trust issue would have been enough to put her on shaky ground.

Sending girls off to college is not merely a promotion to "the thirteenth grade." Like puberty, marriage, and childbirth, college is a "separating point" that requires emotional and mental health to negotiate successfully. When there are unresolved relationship issues creating insecurity between adolescent and parent, or secrets involving traumatic experiences, they usually emerge to damage the next life stage, whatever it may be.

In Lana's case, her "breakdown" took her from being a college freshman in a top-tier college (a strong testament to her intelligence) to a degrading occupation in a trashy environment that promoted drug use.

Preparation for residential college requires a thorough examination of a girl's emotional strengths in addition to academic ability and the declared desire to leave home. Relationships promoting security are vital for all girls. The development of successful adult femininity is a complex and delicate task and cannot withstand many assaults, chief among them sexual abuse, without impairing the outcome. Childhood sexual abuse undermines the best attempts to create that security.

9

Rose:
"I Remember Those
Hairy Arms"

Rose came to therapy at the age of nineteen. She was an attractive girl, dressed in nearly skin-tight clothes that flattered her feminine curves. She had been referred by her physician, who had noticed what Rose later admitted—that she was cutting herself on her forearms and upper thighs.

Rose was born in a Middle Eastern country and had come here as an infant with her parents, both of whom were industrious businesspeople. As their business grew, they helped other members of their families emigrate to the United States. One of these was Rose's father's half-brother Guyan, who came here as a sixteen-year-old when Rose was six. They took him in and gave him a small room off the kitchen.

Rose's parents thought Guyan would make a good babysitter, which they needed since both had to work at the family business full-time. During the first month of babysitting, he was playful when he made her breakfast, took her to school, and picked her up at the end of the school day. As her parents' trust in him grew, they assigned him the additional task of waking her up and helping her get dressed. This way they could leave for work earlier—before Rose awakened.

After a short period of time, Guy (as he wanted to be called, in order to sound more American) began touching Rose inappropriately, pulling her panties up and down to tease her, and generally making getting dressed in the morning a terror for her. She told her mother that she didn't like her uncle and hoped he would move away soon. Her mother explained that they needed him to take care of her because the family business depended on both parents being at work all day. If the business failed, there would not be enough money for them to live on. Rose was intimidated by her mother's explanation, realizing she could not express her protest any more explicitly lest she jeopardize the family unity and make them angry with her. She worried about being sent back to their home country if she was too much trouble.

So Rose became more passive toward her uncle's gestures, and he became more aggressive, sensing he would not be caught or interfered with. Within a month he began to rape her. She remembered the blood, initially, and his frantic cleaning of sheets and washing her clothes. Soon the blood stopped. Her body had adjusted to his body. She began to dissociate, to "leave" her body, becoming oblivious to the events; finally she was able to forget their occurrence completely. Her mind had created a way to get through these days that she thought would go on forever. He did move out after a year. When he visited she always found a way to be out of the house. Though she had lost all memory of the abuse and rapes, she knew she disliked and feared him intensely.

During the first month of therapy Rose complained about being neglected as a child by her parents. She said they thought only about their business and never paid any attention to her except to ask her how she was doing in college. Business was good and Rose had everything she needed—expensive clothing, an expensive car, and lots of spending money. Yet she was angry with her parents and lived in a constant state of fear that she didn't understand.

During the second month of therapy, Rose took a one-week trip to Paris. When she returned she presented me with the news that she had lost her virginity, but she was puzzled because there was no bleeding or discomfort, which her friend had told her to expect.

At the beginning of the third session after her return from Paris, Rose screamed: "His arms—they were hairy! I remember those hairy arms! The hairy arms! The rape! It was my uncle!" Rose was now flooded with memories of her childhood abuse, and for the next twenty minutes was in a state of severe agitation and crying as she explained these events. Then she stopped, stared silently straight ahead for a minute, got up, walked over to a glass-top table covered with seashells, crawled under it, curled herself into a ball facing upward at the glass bottom of the table. She pointed to the seashells and started making humming sounds to herself. She was incoherent. Clearly Rose was now dissociated. I waited for ten minutes, then asked her if she'd like to come out from under the table.

In response she began the journey back from incoherence to reality: with a detached smile on her face she slowly uncurled her body, rolled over, crawled out, and resumed her seat in the chair. "Is our time up?" she asked pleasantly.

I replied that as a matter of fact it was. I further explained that I thought that this was a particularly upsetting session and that I had telephoned her mother while she had been under the table. I told Rose that her mother and father needed to take her to a psychiatric hospital. Both parents arrived at the office, along with her brother. Rose was in a passive, compliant mood and offered no resistance when she was told they were going to take her to a hospital "for a rest."

The defense mechanism of dissociation—that state of mentally blocking out reality—develops in the abused child as protection from incomprehensible and overwhelming pain and terror. It is one of the central mechanisms of coping with trauma. At the time of the traumatic event or events, it is the brain's kindness to the mind, much like fainting from physical pain.

Dissociation not only keeps the child from awareness of the abuse while it is occurring; it also keeps some or all memories of the abuse from consciousness, since remembering trauma can feel like reliving it. Dissociation took over when Rose's forgotten memories surfaced and became unbearably painful for her. Her amnesia from this dissociative episode was so effective that she didn't remember getting under the table or, for that matter, her preceding outburst.

But repeated trauma causes repeated dissociation. Under these circumstances the dissociation can occur with less provocation, for example, when anticipating that a similar abusive situation might become worse. This response turns the once-valuable "anesthetic" into a reaction to many difficult situations (not just sexual abuse) and to fears they might happen. As a result, gaps occur in the person's consciousness and memory which affect her experiences as well as her ability to communicate and sustain relationships. An increasing frequency in dissociated episodes can break down the cohesion of the personality, eventually resulting in a psychotic state.

Some people who suffer from dissociation try to adapt a distant posture with those around them in order to insulate themselves from the sense of vulnerability that might cause them to dissociate. The result is that they come across as cold, perhaps developing a stilted or stylized speech pattern. They may avoid getting close to anyone and remain lonely throughout their lives. If they suffer frequent episodes of dissociation, they may appear "weird" or "crazy" to those who know them. Treating dissociation is a critical aspect of healing the damage done to survivors of childhood sexual abuse. (Of course, this is not to say the development of dissociation is limited to this cause—other kinds of repeated trauma, such as occurs in war, can cause some people to develop a pattern of dissociation.)

After her first voluntary sexual experience prompted her to remember the childhood rapes, Rose was able to recall many more details of the original assaults. Some memories she could handle using rage and tears, while others caused her to dissociate. She tried hard to resolve these memories and feelings and to focus on her adult life. She found herself in dread of another sexual assault, perhaps from a stranger, a neighbor, even a classmate who looked at her a moment too long. She took a martial arts course in self-defense for women, which helped abate some of her fears of assault.

Eventually Rose brought her parents into a therapy session and told them the stories of her abuse. They were horrified. They informed Rose that Guyan had died of cancer so they could not confront him. They apologized for having allowed him to be her babysitter, at the same time indicating they did not imagine what he was capable of doing. This discovery shocked all of them. They knew she was referred to me because she was cutting herself but no one involved (her doctor or me) was looking for evidence of childhood sexual abuse.

Unfortunately, things got worse before they got better. Rose increasingly alternated between episodes of cutting and dissociation, both of which became increasingly serious, dangerous, and frequent. It took one psychiatric hospitalization and years of treatment for these symptoms to diminish. During this period she had nothing to do with men romantically. She was trying to process her residual anger toward her father for his half brother's assaults on her. Her father initially was horrified, but later he became angry with Rose for not forgiving him. She punished him by wasting large sums of money on luxuries, which he could not easily afford. Having remembered the childhood rapes, she was now experiencing a conscious hatred of men.

Rose had chosen a male therapist for several reasons none of which were conscious: The first was to test his ability to deal with her symptoms and help her with her plight. Second, she needed a male therapist with whom she could revise her seductive behavior.

Finally, a male therapist would give her the opportunity to safely and directly express her fear of and rage toward men. Once I had passed all these tests, she would allow me to help her stop dissociating, both in and out of the office, and to stop cutting herself.

Choosing a therapist of the same gender as the abuser, though it may be an unconscious choice, provides an opportunity for the patient to express intense feelings created by the abuse. She can use the therapist as the object of her unresolved feelings toward the abuser. It is the therapist's task to interpret these feelings, and her behavior in therapy, as *transference* on her part: she transfers her fears and anger onto the therapist as if he or she were the abuser. The therapist helps the patient interpret these feelings as rightly "belonging to" (caused by) the abuser only. As the patient gains this insight, she can stop transferring these feelings onto other people who may in one way or another remind her of the perpetrator but who in fact are not abusing her. If this process is successful, she will eventually be freed of the negative legacy of her past.

Another important aspect of this case is the intensity and prevalence with which the patient experienced her flashbacks, which would disrupt her ability to remain in control of her thought process while she relived her painful memories. It was vital for me to be mindful of the pace of therapy; we need to move slowly in order to prevent dissociation. (We will be discussing therapeutic spacing in greater depth in Chapter 29.) At times, Rose had to be brought back from the edge of dissociation with reminders of where she was, using the safe context of therapy to help her cultivate the ability to stay in the present while she addressed painful thoughts and feelings. When she was able to face her traumatic past and deal with her anger about the abuse, she was no longer prone to dissociation.

Rose eventually forgave her parents and warily resumed dating, at first only on a casual basis. During the course of therapy, Rose's cutting diminished and she was able to give it up entirely within a year.

10

Emily:
Cornered

Emily was referred to me for therapy at the age of sixteen suffering from depression, low self-esteem, and self-cutting. This was in the 1970s, when therapists expected to see cutting only among the sickest of mentally ill patients. She was the first patient I treated who cut herself.

Emily grew up in a wealthy section of Manhattan and lived in a luxury apartment house that employed a doorman and elevator operator. She had a younger sister and lived with her parents.

Several weeks into therapy, Emily telephoned me to state in a wooden voice, "I'm calling you because my sister is crying."

"Why is your sister crying?"

"Because I'm cutting my fingers and the bleeding is scaring her."

"Is there anyone else at home?"

"No, I'm babysitting her."

"Can you stop the bleeding with peroxide and Band-Aids, or do the cuts require medical assistance?"

"I think I can do it myself."

"Good, clean up the cuts and call me back after you've calmed your sister."

"Okay."

Since I was inexperienced with self-mutilation, I simply addressed the cutting as a first-aid problem. In future discussions,

I asked her how long this had been going on, if anything triggered the cutting, what she felt when it was happening, and of course, whether the cutting was a suicidal gesture. She didn't seem to know why she was doing it, but she did tell me that she wasn't suicidal.

During a later session she spoke about how going home made her anxious. I asked about her parents and family relationships. None of her answers was remarkable until I asked her about the apartment itself and the building she lived in. Her voice sounded trancelike when she explained that there was a man who operated the elevator. When he took her to or from her apartment on the tenth floor, and there was no one else in the elevator, he would stop it between floors, grab her by her face, and kiss her, thrusting his tongue into her mouth. This would last for a minute or two; then he would restart the elevator and take her to her floor without any mention of what he had just done. I asked her how long this lasted. She told me it had begun when she was seven years old—when her parents deemed her ready to go to school alone—and had stopped when she turned twelve.

Emily confided to her younger sister about the abuse after beginning therapy. They were both surprised to discover that the elevator operator was behaving this way with both of them. After discussing the situation between them, they felt this information would be too troubling to their parents. (Incidentally, sometime later, while Emily and I were preparing for her to make this information known to her parents, the elevator operator was shot to death by a robber in the lobby of her building, making future confrontation of the perpetrator impossible.)

Emily's stress was compounded, however, by the fact that her previous therapist, who treated Emily for anxiety when she was aged twelve to fifteen, suffered from depression herself and committed suicide by jumping out of her tenth-floor office window. This abandonment contributed to Emily's sense of being unprotected, a perception that all abused children feel. Her therapist's suicide contributed to her pessimism and depression in another way as well: because young patients often see their therapists as being like parents, and because children identify with the parent of the same gender, the effect on Emily of having an impaired therapist of the same gender was similar to having an impaired parent: Emily at age fifteen saw little hope for conquering her own problems when the person appointed to help her killed herself.

Emily had shared her problems concerning depression and cutting with both of her parents. Her mother's reaction was to get depressed and frightened. Her father barely reacted at all, probably out of fear he would say the wrong thing. Fear and heartbreak are understandable reactions by parents when they see their child impaired by psychological problems. Emily's parents also lacked information about the cause of these problems; they did not find out about the elevator operator's abuse until she was twenty, eight years after it had stopped. By then, Emily had been dealing with mental and emotional distress for many years. Without the input of a concerned adult, Emily and her sister had decided to keep the abuse a secret.

Often, secrecy regarding sexual abuse is imposed by the abuser, enforced with frightening threats about what he will do to her and her family. In this case, the secrecy was self-imposed, but the effect was the same; it compounded the destructiveness of the abuse. The effects of Emily's assaults manifested themselves in depression, but also in dissociative states that were often accompanied by amnesia.

Emily continued in therapy with me for several years. We were able to resolve the negative consequences of her abuse—revulsion relating to this man's behavior, a fear of being kissed by anyone, her dissociative episodes, depression, and cutting—more quickly than with similar problems in patients who are violated more severely and by members of their own family. Nevertheless, Emily did develop the same symptoms; had these gone untreated, they might have become more entrenched and severe. Then she would have been indistinguishable from survivors whose abuse was worse.

As mentioned earlier, Emily was the first patient I saw who, though generally functional and intact, cut herself. I was able to work with her as an outpatient and thus had the opportunity to understand that self-mutilation is rarely a symptom of suicidal thoughts or severe mental illness. As of this writing, many therapists are still unfamiliar with the reasons for self-mutilation and as a result are reluctant to treat it.

Instead of expressing suicidal intentions, self-mutilation is often a symptom of traumatic childhood events that are highly treatable in effective psychotherapy. By recovering from what seemed at first to be an alarming and hard-to-cure mental illness, Emily provides an example of the mind's potential for health and its response to therapy.

11

Cassie:
The "Phantom Palette"

When Cassie came into treatment with me, she was fifty-two. She presented herself as an incest survivor who until age forty-eight had had no memory of the three-times-a-week episodes of abuse by her father, which occurred from age seven to eleven.

Cassie had been married to the same man for twenty-nine years. Her husband was an unproductive poet, seldom finishing anything he started, and with no source of income besides an occasional small book contract for the last twenty years. He was so unreliable that at times he would not even complete the book he contracted for, and would be asked to return the money advanced to him. Cassie herself had trained to become an artist in college and had been a painter throughout her adult life. She made a little money from her paintings.

To help Cassie and her husband financially, her father gave them a monthly stipend, which sustained them but kept them in "artistic poverty." Intermittently, Cassie's father financed her husband's start-up businesses, all of which failed. Her father was a retired surgeon, well respected in the midwestern city where Cassie grew up. Her mother had been a major philanthropic figure in the community before senility set in.

Cassie and her husband had two children: a son, who would have been twenty-four if still alive, had died of AIDS; a daughter, who was twenty, and was a self-mutilator, primarily a cutter.

Growing up, Cassie had had two brothers. Jack, the elder, developed a neurological disorder that caused severe brain damage, leaving him extremely autistic and violent at the age of five. When he was a child, his parents had taken him to numerous experts, who all pronounced him "hopeless." Cassie also had a younger brother, William, who (as we shall see) was "normal" but later developed his own problems.

Cassie recalled what it was like to grow up with Jack. "Jack would throw temper tantrums at meals. My mother would drag him up one flight of well-kicked wooden stairs. At the top was the room she locked him in until he stopped kicking and screaming. Then she would just come back to the table like nothing had happened. She'd hang the key back on its hook—it actually had a tag that said 'Dungeon' on it. Talking about it now, it's hard to believe, but it's true. We lived like that for three years."

She described her home as "spooky; yes, that's how it felt. Lots of strange things went on there, and neither of my parents explained anything to us. We—my brother and I—never even talked to each other about what we saw or what we thought about it. I always worried that I would be put in the room locked with the 'dungeon' key. When Jack was sent away to the asylum, I wondered if either of us would be next. I don't know to this day what my brothers thought. The lack of talk in the house was a deafening silence, like music in a horror movie. I believed that if I ever . . . ever told my mother what my father was doing to me—and I didn't even know it was called rape—the dungeon would be waiting for me. It was unthinkable for me to have any judgmental ideas about my family or our household. I got very good at not remembering anything that happened at home that was questionable. There was just this eerie feeling that overcame you when you walked in the door, even if no one was in the house. It was such a big, old stone Tudor that it would take a few minutes to be able to tell who was there, if anybody. Remember, we were young and little, and the house was large even by adult standards. To us it was a haunted castle. Dr. Whitelaw—that's how we all referred to my father—demanded quiet at every meal, and quiet was the hallmark and terror of my family's house."

Cassie continued, "Anyway, I guess Jack got too big for my mother to handle, so they sent him away. We would visit him on Sundays after church. We would drive two hours to this strange building surrounded by a fence with barbed wire on top. We would walk through the giant main entrance, and above the door, carved in stone it said State Asylum for the Insane.

"I didn't know what that meant, but I just assumed it meant people like Jack. We would take turns talking to Jack, but he acted like he didn't know who we were or what we were saying. He didn't even look at us most of the time. I think we each made up things he was thinking so the visits would have meaning for us."

Jack had been institutionalized at the age of eight; adults were housed with children at this hospital, and at the age of fourteen he was murdered by an adult patient. "Dr. Whitelaw had Jack's remains cremated and sprinkled the ashes in his rose garden," Cassie went on. Even in therapy sessions, so many years after these events, she never called him Dad or Father—always Dr. Whitelaw. "I was four when Jack was 'struck with the fever' [the brain damage that caused his autism]. My younger brother, William, was two at the time, and he was nine at the time of Jack's death. He protested scattering Jack's ashes in the rose garden. William hated that garden for all the times the thorns scratched him. Anyway, my little brother grew up to be severely alcoholic. He drank himself to death by his fortieth birthday. When William died, Dr. Whitelaw scattered his ashes on the same roses—for fertilizer. I wondered why Dr. Whitelaw and William seemed to . . . almost hate each other for so many years. But as I said, no one talked to each other in my family."

■

With this introduction to Cassie's background and family history, let's take a closer look at her therapy beginning with her first session with me. When Cassie entered my office, she was the very picture of a conservative middle-aged matron: She dressed conservatively in a wool tweed suit. Her hair was curly and short. She wore horn-rimmed glasses. Her manner of speaking was clear and direct. "I've come here because I have many issues from my childhood that have affected my behavior throughout my life, damaging my family, at times [causing me to] neglect my children. I have been in therapy for two years, but I feel I have skirted all these issues and want to start again."

As she spoke, her individual facial features contradicted each other: her eyes looked terrified while her mouth maintained a small smile. She spoke almost matter-of-factly, in the sort of detached tone rape victims often use to describe their experiences to the police.

"Since you seem so clear about your goals, why don't you tell me what these issues are?"

"From the time I was seven until I was twelve, my father would come into my bedroom in the middle of the night, wake me up, and rape me. The first time he did this, he put his hand over my mouth and said, 'Be a big girl now. Don't be a baby.' This terrified me. I could hardly breathe between his weight on top of me and the size of his penis inside of me. After a while my body stretched to accommodate his penis even though I was so young and small. The terror and pain never did go away during those years, but somehow when he was finished, walked out, and closed my bedroom door, it was like it never happened. I forgot every episode completely until four years ago. I had thirty-six years of amnesia."

Her deliberate manner in telling this story was striking. I asked if she understood why she had forgotten these traumatic memories and why she remembered them when she did.

She shook her head and raised her eyebrows in mild reproach, but she responded articulately. "My father was the most respected man in the city. He had saved many lives. He spent time with me and taught me about butterflies, birds, and entomology. He taught me how to ice skate, sail our boat, ski, and took me hiking. He was my teacher and expressed interest in me and my development, though he managed to express this interest without warmth. I guess if I had remembered what he did to me, I would have had to lose any connection to him. How could I enjoy all the things that we did together during the day, all the things he taught me, and the privilege of being Dr. Whitelaw's daughter? I guess it was more important not to lose 'the good daddy' than to find a way to make him stop raping me. In time, I imagine I thought of him as my lover. I had to put him in some context, though I never remembered the sex, just had a vague sense of secret romance. In a strange way I felt very special to him."

Cassie exhibited unusual confidence telling this story; there was no embarrassment or apology in her presentation. She had answered the first part of my question without skipping a beat, then went on to address the second half of my question: "As to how I came to remember these events, well, I am a landscape painter. I always have been. One day I started to paint cows into my landscapes. My change of subject surprised me, but you know how a novel can write itself? Well, so can a painting develop a direction of its own that the painter follows. Gradually, I noticed that the faces of the cows were beginning to look more and more like my mother. I felt like I was painting ghosts that had inhabited my mind for a very long time, as if I was using a phantom palette . . . First, inklings came to me, then all the memories descended in a torrent. When I realized what had happened, I became angry with my mother, not my father. You see, I remembered that she allowed him to move his twin bed away from hers and put it along the wall that ended at [their bedroom] door, making it easier for him to slip out without disturbing her. What could she have been thinking?"

Cassie told her story in a low voice, devoid of drama and interlaced with pauses. "After the memories returned, I thought he must have been crazy, but even so, *she* should have protected me from his craziness. Of course, no one challenged Dr. Whitelaw and he never communicated personally to anyone, including my mother. He was a mystery to all of us, and we took that for granted.

I have called him 'Dr. Whitelaw' my whole life, never 'Daddy' or 'Dad.' I think my mother called him that in front of us children, though I overheard her call him 'Vern' (for Vernon) when they were alone or thought they were."

She offered another example of her father's emotional distance. "Once he and I were out sailing; there were other small sailboats nearby and I was his only crew. I approached him to give him a hug. He pushed me away and said 'Not here,' but where could I hug him? He was unapproachable, even though he could approach you and rape you."

"You mentioned that you are unresolved about many issues, yet you tell this story in a manner that suggests you *have* thought about and resolved them. I am curious about the terrified look on your eyes in contrast to the smile on your mouth as you tell me all this."

"That's the look of a little girl about to be raped by her father, and it never leaves my face. I guess there must be lots of issues, at least partially hidden, to resolve."

"So we have Little Cassie and Grown-up Cassie living in continuous disharmony in your head."

"I like that description. I want Little Cassie out of my head."

"Well, I guess we have established one of our goals for treatment."

Cassie came in to her second session quite animated. "I didn't forget what you said during our last session. I've been thinking a lot about all the ways that Little Cassie inhabits my mind. The major one is sexual. She has me looking at men and planning their seduction. And although I don't act on it, I still consider walking over and beginning my dance of seduction. I may be fifty-two, but I can tell by how men look at me that I have the ability to attract them and drag them off to bed. So I have to stop Little Cassie from acting on the impulse. I don't even want to have these fantasies. That might just make me act on them [again], and I don't want to."

Throughout her marriage, Cassie had cheated on her husband. When he first discovered this, he reacted by cheating as well, sometimes with the wife of the man Cassie was cheating with in their bohemian crowd. This kind of reciprocal cheating went on for years, at almost every opportunity, until the frequency of mutual cheating became so great that they could no longer keep score. It became their marital style, which lasted until their daughter attempted suicide. Aware of what was going on, she had a breakdown, in which she nearly took her life. Her attempted suicide is what drove Cassie into therapy with her first therapist.

"You don't want this to happen because of the possible consequences to your marriage?"

"Partially, but more because when I'm Little Cassie I always feel like I'm being raped even if I'm in charge and the initiator. I'm tired of feeling like that, but it's still a struggle. I always feel like I'm getting fucked, physically and metaphorically."

"Do you like to curse?"

"I love it if it's descriptive of what I've gone through. . . . I don't want to pretty up any of this. It's very ugly and its consequences have put me in indefensible situations with men, their wives, our friends, and of course my husband, and it hasn't died down completely. Even though I stopped cheating, he is always suspicious when I leave the house. He still screams at me; he calls me a whore, a slut, and anything else he can think of, although I haven't acted on Little Cassie's commands for a few years now. Sid's twelve years older than me, has had a few strokes along with diabetes, and although he's not good in bed anymore, that has nothing to do with my impulses. I mean, he used to be a great lover, but that never stopped me. Anyway, he's not about to get even with me like he used to. But he's still bitter. He can just scream.

"I think his refusal to earn enough money for us to live was always his way of getting even with me. We're squatters, you know. We live in an old warehouse in the Village, where we steal electricity for heat and light along with about twenty others who have carved apartments for themselves out of loft space. I don't think my daughter even knows what we've been doing, even after ten years of this, although I guess on some level children know everything. She cuts herself with razor blades while she's getting As in school.

She talks to a social worker at her school who knows we're broke. We have serious money troubles, but part of me feels like I deserve the poverty."

"Do you feel you deserve it for the infidelities?"

"No, because I stole my father from my mother."

As a result of her relationship with her father, Cassie had become an "Oedipal winner." The *Oedipus complex*, first described by Sigmund Freud, is the process whereby children develop a sense of gender and sexual identity. The first man in a girl's life is her father. She is drawn to him as her hero and protector, someone who makes her feel special because she is a girl. This is a childlike romance: in a normal, affectionate father-daughter relationship, it will help her learn to appreciate her femininity, so that during puberty she can become attracted to boys.

In a healthy Oedipal complex, this affectionate relationship with her father starts in late infancy and develops over the next five to six years. After that it becomes latent or hidden, reappearing in its adolescent form when the girl develops romantic crushes on boys, no longer her father. Some fathers prize masculinity so greatly that the daughter may develop masculine traits and tastes in athletics, dress, gait, and general personality styles to paradoxically "romance her father" in a nonsexual way.

In the case of father-daughter rape or other incestuous activities, the daughter's Oedipal stage as a true sexual partner is literally consummated, which causes her a great sense of guilt regarding her mother as well as sexual attraction toward her father. These feelings are usually unconscious in the girl, but often can be inferred from her behavior—sexual aggression or avoidance, self-destructive behaviors, self-loathing, or other issues. Cassie chose sexual aggression in the form of promiscuously cheating on her husband.

"Would you like to have your husband here for a session? Maybe you need to express how you feel about the current state of both the relationship and the household finances."

Cassie broke into a big smile. "Yes, I think that would give me a chance to settle up with him, since I can't with the other man in my life, Dr. Whitelaw."

On the day of the joint session, Sid came into the office first, sporting an expensive-looking cane that he actually needed to steady himself since his last stroke. He looked around the room. "Nice paintings."

"My wife's the painter."

"Yours too?" he asked.

"Yes."

"Tough crew, these women painters . . ."

"Tougher than men painters?"

"Nah, I guess not."

"Do I take your comments to mean that your relationship with Cassie is 'tough'?"

Cassie sat down on the couch next to Sid.

"Better than it used to be. Less lying, I hope, less arguing."

"Sid . . . you still scream at me all the time."

Sid didn't respond.

"Cassie, would you like to see a change in Sid's behavior?"

"Sure—less lying deserves less screaming, right?"

"Maybe if you stopped nagging at me about money . . . ! You just don't give it a rest! You know I have a big book deal in the works!"

Cassie just looked at him and rolled her eyes.

"I hear you've had a tough time in the publishing world," I commented.

He nodded and stroked his white beard. "To be fair, I've given that world a hard time." He gave a little laugh while his wife glumly shook her head.

Despite Cassie's eye rolling I decided to pursue the income issue. "How did you give them a hard time?"

"Made a lot of promises I didn't deliver on, keeping book advances for work I never finished. . . . Cassie here is doing all right for herself: Whitelaw money bailed us all out. She won't let me touch it. I don't even know where it is or how much there is."

"Why is that?"

"Probably it's because people give me a lot of trouble when it comes to money—"

"No, Sid," Cassie interrupted. "You've just stolen too much from us . . . and just about everybody you've dealt with."

"I think I've just been too nice a guy, Cassie."

"No dear, you've been too much of a rat."

Sid looked surprised, then broke into a smile and started laughing. "Yes, maybe that's more accurate."

We had several more couples sessions, which gave them both an opportunity to discuss old grievances and work on new ways to communicate. Though most of their marriage had been something of a calamity, they still had warm feelings for each other and, like other older couples I have worked with, they had the capacity to heal some old wounds. Years of infidelity, however, had taken a great toll on their relationship. Because of their long history of dysfunction, they did not do as well as couples who seek help at the start of their marital difficulties.

Several months later Cassie told me about the incest survivor group she was attending to enhance her individual therapy. This was helping her in many ways, including expanding the ways she looked at her abuse. "There is never only one way to view it for any of us. We've all got our demons, or Little Cassie's—the fucked parts of us. It was relieving to hear the horrible experiences that the other women went through. It meant I wasn't alone anymore. I wasn't a freak . . ."

Support groups are especially helpful for problems that involve secrecy and shame. There is a valuable transition from being a social pariah to a member of a social alliance, where people are encouraged to unburden their most troubling thoughts and feelings among people with similar histories.

"I've noticed in recent months as we've been talking that your eyes don't look terrified any longer and your expressiveness is far more varied."

She smiled. "Yes, I had to get a new pair of glasses that don't have to cover bulging eyes with raised eyebrows. Little Cassie is getting weaker, losing her voice."

After two years of therapy Cassie walked into my office and stated flatly, "Well, the bastard's dead. And there's an inheritance. He made it to ninety-three, continually checking his pulse, monitoring his own dying. You could see him sitting there in the parlor mumbling numbers, his diminishing pulse rate. But he never acknowledged what he'd done to me and to my brother William. I think after all is said and done, I hate him most for taking all his secrets to his grave. It's ironic, I married a man who wouldn't support me and my father had to give me money for his whole life and afterward. I guess I always had two men—one legitimate, the other my secret crime. Well, my husband's not yelling at me anymore. I don't have to pray that he'll finish a book or follow through on a hairbrained business scheme he promises will get us out of having to live like thieves. No more squatting! I'm going apartment hunting."

Cassie was free of Little Cassie completely after about four years of therapy. She was fifty-six at the time. I wanted to ask her if she regretted the forty-four years of being dominated by incest. I didn't ask, but she must have intuited my question because she smiled and said, "I don't know how many years I've got left, but they'll be without Little Cassie and the incest man, and that will be enough."

Cassie continued coming to treatment and for the most part talked about issues of lesser importance. Every once in a while, however, she sensed a Little Cassie impulse and discussed it with a smile, knowing she wasn't tempted. She continued this lighter therapy until she was sixty-one. She didn't want to relinquish the conversations that had begun as her bridge out of hell.

Father-daughter incest is probably the most destructive form of the sexual abuses in terms of the extent of psychological damage—often lasting throughout the daughter's life and producing the greatest number of psychological disorders and behaviors. These include dissociation, amnesia, self-loathing, self-injury, anorexia, phobias, provocation of assault or rape by other men, compulsive promiscuity, revulsion relating to any sexual activities, and psychotic episodes. In Cassie's case, incest profoundly affected her as well as her marriage and her children.

Cassie's abuse had caused her massive confusion throughout her childhood. On an unconscious level she felt the fear, pain, and terror her father was inflicting on her. On a conscious level, she had to adapt to this ongoing situation and keep herself together. She didn't want to lose her relationship with her father and all the benefits that came with it. Her emotional task was to find it morally acceptable and develop behaviors that proved it so to her. She became sexually promiscuous as soon as her father stopped his abusive behavior, thereby continuing to legitimize what her father had done to her. During adolescence she needed to see herself as desirable and tempting to as many boys as possible. This kept her sense of identity intact.

Cassie stayed away from close friendships with girls since she feared their anger the same way she feared what she assumed would be her mother's anger toward her if she knew Cassie had been more of a wife (sexually) to her father than her mother had been. Since her abuse had begun at an Oedipal age, Cassie saw this as a special recognition of her by her father. She was able to view it this way because she had gradually adjusted physically and psychologically to his assaults.

In adulthood her adjustments and behaviors were increasingly viewed as inappropriate because they threatened all her relationships. They were no longer helpful or productive to Cassie and so had become obsolete, like many a child's adjustments to abuse, neglect, and family dysfunction. In Cassie's case, she was a committed painter; it was her art—her phantom palette—that brought her memories back so she could begin to change these damaging adjustments she had made during an abnormal childhood.

12

Olivia:
The Effect of Sexual
Abuse on Marriage

Olivia entered treatment in her early thirties. Her complaint was her total disinterest in any form of sex. She had no sexual desire at all and lacked the ability to be aroused. During her marriage she had complied when her husband wanted to have sex, but he sensed her reluctance. After several years of marriage he told her he was tired of always being the one asking for sex, and he wanted a divorce. By the time she came to treatment, at the suggestion of her gynecologist, they had been divorced for a year. She had custody of her two sons, four and two years old.

In early sessions Olivia spoke very softly and seemed mildly depressed. In her second session she told me about the suicide of a close woman friend, a prominent sculptor who had talked frequently about not wanting to live before she actually took her life. Witnessing her friend's slow unstoppable descent into suicide had taken a toll on Olivia. We talked about this for several sessions before she began a narration about her own sadness, starting with her childhood. She had distinct memories of wanting to be a cripple. When she was ten years old, she borrowed a pair of crutches from a friend and on weekends walked around the house using them.

Olivia also talked about her concern, during the marriage, of leaving her husband alone with their children. She was afraid that he would molest them, though there had never been any incidents or complaints from her boys.

"Was there anyone in your home when you were a child who molested you?"

"Yes, my father." She stared at the floor. "He did that a lot. He had me lie across his thighs on my stomach and he penetrated me. After the third time, I would grab a book and read it, concentrating intensely, so intensely that I couldn't feel anything down there. I can honestly say that after a while I had no idea what he was doing to me. I was numb, as numb as you get from dental novocaine. He did the same thing to my younger sister a few years later. He continued abusing her until she was fifteen. She went to the school authorities about him and promptly had a nervous breakdown. She once told me that he could bring her to orgasm. She went away to boarding school and never spoke to him again. The boarding school was the recommendation of the court. The judge gave him a choice between that and having her put in a foster home."

"Your sister had a nervous breakdown; it's not surprising. This is a brutal experience for a child to endure." Olivia remained stoically calm. I went on. "How are you now? Did your father's actions create a lasting effect on you?"

"Well, that anesthesia—the 'novocaine' I developed—along with the ability to 'disappear' and leave my numb body behind hasn't gone away. I have no ability to change this. When my husband and I were dating, I tried to experience our 'making out' the same way my friends told me they did—that it was exciting. I faked it all. When I saw my ob-gyn for the first time, he was solicitous and I guess gentle when he examined me, but it didn't matter because I couldn't feel anything anyway. It's permanent. My brain and genitals are not connected."

"Do you want them to be?"

"I think so but I'm not sure. I want to enjoy sexual pleasure but there's something secure about the separation. What I don't like about it is that I have no control over it. I can't get excited or aroused. There are times when I definitely want to experience those feelings. Sometimes I meet a man and I want to have a full experience with him, but I can't will the sensations to return or the numbness to go away."

"Have you ever discussed what happened to you with your mother?"

"I watched my sister discuss this with my mother. I was very discouraged. My mother seemed to be in a dream world that let her be detached from my sister—and this was while the case was in court! There seemed to be no point."

I invited Olivia's mother in for a session. After exchanging pleasantries with this very expensively dressed, made-up, and coiffed woman, I asked her, "Does it disturb you that your husband sexually abused two of your three daughters?" (Olivia's youngest sister had run away to boarding school while her middle sister's case was pending in court.) Her mother looked at me with a broad, wide-eyed smile and responded, "Why—don't all daddies do that?"

I was so dumbstruck (and at the time inexperienced) that I failed to ask her if her own father had sexually abused her as a child. Whether or not this had happened, perhaps she chose not to see what was happening to her daughters in order to avoid finding fault with her parenting or her marriage, thereby keeping the marriage intact. Her husband was, after all, a very wealthy and influential man. Although I did not pursue the question of what motivated her "dream world," I had just glimpsed it firsthand.

Olivia had had no opportunity to share with her mother what had happened to her as a child; worse than that, as Olivia revealed in an earlier, individual session, she had concluded from witnessing her mother's reaction to her sister that her own disclosure of abuse would be met by cold detachment. Olivia needed a *therapeutic alliance*, a relationship with a skilled helper whom she trusted, in order to talk explicitly about her father. She needed to complain, to cry, and hear someone say what her mother could not—that her father was wrong in abusing his daughters.

Therapy helped her address her unspoken certainty that all men were predators, that all fathers were molesters. Her sexuality had been frozen in childhood by the abuse. Returning to it verbally allowed her to express the feelings of hurt, anger, and fear that had become bound together with her sexual feelings, blocking them all with emotional novocaine.

Throughout her several years in treatment (aged thirty-two to thirty-five), she remained low-key and shy. This was in contrast to many survivors of abuse, who describe the violations they endured with volume and often vulgarity as if to assure themselves and others that they will never be silent victims again. Olivia's quiet demeanor, however, did not prevent her from changing her life for the better. Gradually, the broken connection between her will and her sexuality mended. After dating several men, she married one of them. When she got a job with a large corporation in their security department, she was ahead of her time, glass ceiling and all, succeeding in an unusual line of work for a woman in that era. She had hundreds of armed security guards under her supervision, an ironic contrast to her timid and traumatic childhood.

Marriage is likely to be jeopardized when one spouse has been sexually molested in childhood. That jeopardy is greater if there has been no disclosure to the other partner; their sexual relationship has to be affected negatively in these circumstances. Olivia's husband left her after five years of marriage because, as he put it, "I'm tired of being a sexual beggar. Your total lack of desire and your passive martyr posture, when you 'do me a favor' by having sex, leaves me with two choices: resign myself to a sexless life, or a sexless marriage in which I turn to another woman or women who will be sexually responsive to me. I don't want to live as a liar and cheat, so I have to choose a third alternative, divorce."

He had no idea that her father had molested her for years. She had never told him. It is critical to the success of a marriage that each individual's personal history of sexual abuse—where it exists—be disclosed, if possible prior to marriage. The couple may then go for counseling to understand how such abuse might affect their sexual relationship before it actually does. Too often it doesn't show up until after they are married.

I have seen several couples in therapy whose sexual relationships throughout courtship were affectionate and successful but which changed abruptly after marriage. While the couples spent the first years of their marriage working out their sexual relationships, including discussions of fragmented flashbacks, we never came to any definite conclusions about why everything seemed all right until after they were married.

However, I believe the problem stems from the phenomenon I call "the forever factor," which comes into play unconsciously when marriage reminds the new wife of her childhood feelings of "permanent sexual captivity" at the hands of her father, brother, uncle, or other male abuser. Perhaps she has chosen her husband for healthy, loving reasons, yet after the wedding vows are spoken, the unconscious association surfaces. Suddenly, to the surprise of both partners, the wife is terrified of her husband and repelled by him sexually.

In some cases the wives develop anorexia and become quite emaciated. During the course of individual therapy and marital counseling, the wife in these cases needs to separate her earlier victimization by her abuser from the relationship she is developing with her husband. She also needs to use therapy to come to terms with the complex meanings of her anorexia, the most physically obvious being the message to the husband, "Look, I'm not a woman —I'm not desirable." Marriage is also strained by the other aspects of anorexia, which include the wife's feelings of lack of entitlement, anxiety, and confusion over emotional needs.

Another ineffective solution to the "problem" of sex in marriage is for the survivor of childhood sexual abuse not to avoid sex but rather to become very aggressive about it, as we saw with Cassie in Chapter 11. Her aggression took the form of cheating on her husband with nearly every man she met, and he in turn cheated on her to get even.

Survivors of childhood sexual abuse understandably feel that they are only valued for their physical selves. Marriage had brought a challenging new dimension to individual therapy for these women: could they overcome the physical and emotional legacy of their abuse? Marital sessions I conducted with these couples gave the husband the opportunity to express his needs as well and to emphasize his concern for his wife's feelings. Conversely, by listening to her story and her needs, counseling helped the wife revise her obsolete feelings and appreciate the reality of her spouse's affection. Talking exercises were developed in which each spouse could ask the other "Who are you?" "What is our current relationship?" These exerecises also helped each partner to stay in the present.

13

Audrey:
The Father

A udrey was twenty-five when she came to treatment. She was a short, curvaceous young woman whose outfit revealed cleavage to the edge of acceptability. She expressed herself with intensity, speaking loudly and rapidly. Her speech was laced with curse words in virtually every sentence she spoke. During most of our sessions, she was irritable, angry, and cried intensely. She was having a great deal of difficulty adjusting to her loss of status due to dismissal by her former employer, a famous philanthropist.

For seven years, she had worked as the philanthropist's nanny. Often she would act toward others as if she were his private secretary. This would cause them to behave deferentially toward her, giving her an artificially elevated sense of importance. She became part of his family, getting involved in family disputes. Finally the philanthropist fired her because she lied to him about using his car.

When Audrey was fired, her self-esteem plummeted. Her former employer, the philanthropist, referred her to therapy. She would get into vituperative arguments with drivers over parking spaces. She had to move home to live with her mother. She found that after years of room, board, and a good salary in a Park Avenue mansion on Manhattan's Upper East Side, she could not accept being an ordinary person with ordinary status.

She tried various skill-training programs ranging from learning computers to learning to be a private physical trainer. She quit them all. She became a telephone solicitor for the sale of illegal drugs. It paid well because of the risk, but she met unsavory and abusive men. She got romantically involved with several of them. This depressed her further, so she self-medicated with marijuana.

She explained her reasons for coming to therapy: "I came here because ever since I dropped out of high school at sixteen, when my father left the house, I have been making one bad decision after another with regard to work, men, friends, and drugs. I've tried a lot of different jobs, started a bunch of projects, but nothing I do lasts for very long. I quit or I'm fired, usually for lying or screwing up. My mother's sick—I think she's dying—and my brother's a junkie. My father never grew up. He rides a Harley and thinks he's a kid at fifty. So I have nobody to look up to. Oh, one small detail. My father molested the hell out of me from the time I was three. I was scared to tell anyone, but when he left us, I accused him of it after he stopped paying child support or any kind of support to my mother. He had the balls to deny it! I've accused him repeatedly. He continues to deny it, but he started sending my mother money again. Isn't that an interesting coincidence?"

"Your former employer gave you status and financial security after your father left your mother. Was he a father figure to you? Was *he* ever inappropriate sexually or any other way with you?"

"No, never. I think that's why I felt so safe there. He was the right kind of fatherly. I feel like he was the kind of father a girl should have. I guess I took too much for granted only to find out that he wouldn't put up with the crap from me that a real father would. I acted out and he fired me. If he was my real father, he'd just be angry or aggravated with me, but he'd be stuck with me. He sure wasn't stuck with me."

"Are you often angry?"

"I'm always angry."

"At who?"

"At everybody, but mostly at myself."

"Why?"

She took a deep breath, but before she could start talking, she started crying. She tried to talk through her sobs, but they were so intense I had to ask her to try to bring them under control so I could understand what she was saying. Glaring at the floor she blurted out, "My father was the only one who could bring me to orgasm!" She then broke down, weeping.

"So this is what makes you angry at yourself?"

"Yes, I should've fought him—I mean I should have felt repulsed, not excited."

"Audrey, you were a small child when he started to molest you. This was not your fault in any way, nor was your physical response."

"But it didn't change when I grew up. It's like he stole my whole sex life. Nobody else even excites me. I keep trying to find a guy who will 'top' him." Her voice thinned to a hissing whisper. Her fists were clenched tightly.

Audrey was angry with most men. She anticipated being abused before they even said hello. Ironically, it was the men who seemed most helpless—the lost boy type—who took advantage of her. She perceived these men as confused and brooding, which made them less threatening to her. They brought out her maternal instincts, causing her to drop her guard. She would then feel she was on a mission to save the man she happened to be sexually attracted to.

For months of sessions, Audrey would express herself with rage-ful crying, sad crying, and much of the time she digressed to the point of incoherence.

"I'm going to ask you to try to do the opposite of what I ask most patients to do. You are very expressive, from sobbing to shouting to cursing. I don't think this is productive for you. You've gone beyond venting pent-up feelings, and now you seem stuck in this behavior. I suspect you do this with many people, including your father and mother, as well as your boyfriends. In my opinion it makes you feel more chaotic, causing you to lose faith in your ability to become stronger and cope. One reason you've become stuck is that your nervous system is in bad shape. You are in too much pain. You are medicating yourself with marijuana. We have better medications

than that. I'm sending you to a psychiatrist to evaluate what medication will be helpful to you. We will work on getting you emotionally ready to look for a legitimate job, so you won't feel like an
outcast."

I was relieved to see that Audrey did not misunderstand my
directive tone as a scolding.

"Yeah, I guess you're right. But my problem is, I can promise to
do what you say now, and by tomorrow my resolve is gone and I'm
high again. As for the 'normal' job, I don't feel like a normal person. I mean, I had sex with my father, so now I guess I feel too
much like an outlaw to belong anywhere. Maybe, if I could get a
job that included the glamor and power I tried to convince myself
and others I once had when I was really only a glorified nanny . . ."

"So you're still having a hard time with the reality of your current situation?"

"My current situation is unbearable! That's why I like to stay
high."

Months went by during which Audrey would tell me she was
looking into training programs, but no matter what program she
applied for, she had a different reason for not going. She continued
to work sporadically, answering telephones for illegal businesses.
When I asked her why she preferred to do that instead of finding a
legitimate job, she explained, "Because I'm off the books, it does-
n't screw up my social security benefits, I don't pay taxes, and most
importantly, it pays twenty-five dollars an hour, which is more than
I can get anywhere else. I told you that my father denies molesting
me and that he gives my mother some money. What I haven't said
is, it's not enough money to keep food in the house or pay the rent
on her rent-controlled apartment. So I have to earn the most
money I can or we don't eat sometimes."

Needless to say, this stress in matters of everyday survival only
compounded Audrey's anxiety and depression.

Although Audrey did not get the much-needed acknowledgment
or apology from her father, her digressions off the topic diminished
greatly in our sessions. She substituted prescribed medication for

marijuana. She became better at evaluating people and making decisions on a day-to-day basis. But her financial and vocational situation remained unresolved; her longing for the glory days with the philanthropist's family was mixed with shame over her sexual abuse. When the job-training issue came up about two years after we started working together, she slowly began skipping appointments until she had dropped out of treatment entirely.

Six months after her last appointment, she left a message on my voice-mail stating, "I know I have mental illness to a serious degree. I am working with a psychiatrist and hope that through medication I can get myself to the point we had agreed on. Thanks for your help."

I was glad to hear that she was pursuing her recovery, but I have not learned whether her approach of relying primarily on the use of medication was fully successful.

Audrey's life went into crisis when she was forced to make an adjustment to an extreme change in lifestyle after being fired. This was especially difficult for her because the status she gained while working for an important man served as emotional compensation for her childhood abuse, a painful grievance that was never addressed. When she lost her job, she was confronted with her own rage and lack of self-esteem, which drove her to a drug habit and a series of illegal jobs. This shift in lifestyle left her embattled on many fronts: her lack of career preparation, her financial problems, and of course the sexual abuse that had shaped her childhood. She needed support to resolve all of these problems, which had fed on one another and contributed to her illegal drug use. My hope for Audrey is that she has persisted in her struggle to reclaim her life.

14

Ava:
"Poor Kid in a Rich Family"

Ava, an attractive nineteen-year-old, came to therapy for bulimia nervosa. Twenty minutes after ingesting food she would secretly use ipecac, which induces painful, intense, uncontrollable vomiting for about forty-five minutes and causes long-term muscle damage. She also had moderate symptoms of anorexia; at five feet five she weighed just one hundred and five pounds and declared that she wanted to lose more weight. In addition, she had obsessive-compulsive disorder (OCD): she washed frequently to counter her fear of contamination by germs. Her attitude about therapy from the outset seemed positive: she had moved to New York City—about a thousand miles away from home and family—in order to get treatment. Her family was wealthy, so paying for her move and therapy sessions would not present a financial hardship.

Ava had been brought up by a loving nanny, a father who kept to himself, and a mother who provided well for the family. However, her mother had always been preoccupied by the business empire she had inherited. Moreover, Ava stressed, her mother had only male friends and colleagues, and had little use for women. Ava didn't know how she herself fit into the family, and there was a hint of the "damsel in distress" in her manner.

"I feel like I'm my nanny's daughter. Since my parents are rich, with a long lineage in our city, I'm supposed to be a debutante, but the woman who brought me up, my nanny, is lowly in terms of society. So it's like I'm the poor kid in the rich family. It would be dangerous for me to depend on my nanny since she could never defend me against my parents. I always knew that. At the same time she was the only person I could emotionally lean on. Since my mother always talked about women her own age as 'lazy and stupid,' I didn't know whether I could get her to see me as someone she could respect. . . . I didn't think so. I tried all kinds of things to please my mother. I tried to get thin, and I still feel guilty if I'm not losing weight. If I can't exercise enough, I take a bottle of ipecac and puke my guts up after a meal. When all else fails I use cocaine; it kills my appetite. It used to get me high, but now I take it just to avoid the craving—it won't make me high, but if I stop taking it I feel low enough to want to kill myself."

After taking more family history I worked on developing with her the trust and rapport necessary to establish a therapeutic alliance. I addressed some of Ava's complaints. "You have a lot of reasons to feel unhappy, between your confusing position in your family and the desperate failed steps you have taken to try to feel better."

"But I don't know what else to do. I also have a lot of trouble with men. They're pushy with me sexually. I've been groped too often, not romantically but more like my breasts were grapefruits they were squeezing till it hurt, or they're reaching into my pants to poke me rather than romance me or even stimulate me. I always feel like men are attacking me. I have been raped twice."

"Did you go to the police?"

"And have my mother find out? She'd just say I was a whore who deserved it. 'It must be your fault' is all I'd get." Ava became quiet for a moment, then asked haltingly, "Do I dress like a whore? Does it look like I'm asking for it?"

"It's hard to know where to draw the line. Years ago your outfit and the way it fits you would probably have been seen as crossing the line, but today many young women dress to be appealing and sexy beyond old norms. I do see seductive, inviting, and helpless behavior in you that would tempt someone who wanted power over you, maybe sexual power. There are aspects of you that come off as a sexual target. I don't think its ignorance on your part about how to behave. I think you have a need to elicit feelings in men whether you like them or not. I don't think you have much control over it. Can you remember the first time anyone ever molested you sexually?"

Ava became quiet. She looked like she didn't want to answer the question. After a few minutes she spoke in a low voice, "My father had this belt buckle, a big cowboy belt buckle; he would use it on me in ways that hurt. He would use it like an instrument to hurt me down there. He looked like he was having a good time. I could tell he was getting aroused. He would always tell me it was because I had been a bad girl and this was my punishment. It wasn't my punishment. It was his pleasure. It took me years to figure that out. I was three when he started and about seven when he stopped. During those years he thought of other ways to hurt me that excited him. I just don't want to say what they were."

"Ava, it's not necessary to say what they were."

"But I'm afraid you'll think that it's my fault somehow and I deserve what I get from men. Do you think I deserved what I got from my father? That's how my mother thinks."

"No, I don't think you deserve what you get from men. I think that *you* believe, and have always believed, that you deserved what you got from your father. Children don't have the ability to disbelieve their parents. I also think your mother has no idea what your father did to you and would have disapproved of it, to put it mildly."

Ava looked shocked at my interpretation. "You don't think he had her support for all those things he did to me?"

"I can see how he suggested to you that he did and that as a three-year-old you believed him. Do you want to tell your mother now?"

"I just think she won't believe me. I'm not even sure she likes me."

"Do you want to find out?"

"Will you tell her that you believe me?"

"Yes, I do believe you, and I will support your recollections."

At our next session Ava reported that she had told her mother in great detail about the abuse. Her mother said that she found it upsetting but not surprising since she was suspicious of infidelities on his part. One week later Ava's mother accused her father of this behavior. He denied it, unconvincingly according to her mother, who threw him out of the house and started divorce proceedings.

Being believed by her mother had a positive effect on Ava; she felt that her grievances against her father had been somewhat redressed. However, she was still left with the legacy of years of abuse—seventeen years of not being able to tell anyone about it or deal with it constructively—that had shaped her personality. She had developed anorexia, bulimia, OCD, and a seductive, masochistic personality disorder that resulted in her being repeatedly harmed by men. She had also become a cocaine addict in a self-medicating attempt to make some of her psychic pain go away. It would take extensive therapy to treat each harmful effect and disorder resulting from her childhood sexual abuse.

Ava volunteered to go into the rehab division of a hospital to get the cocaine out of her system. She also needed to be evaluated for muscle damage from the ipecac and to get a general checkup to see whether she was taking additional substances she had not disclosed. During her three-month inpatient treatment, she began to solidify new patterns of living without purging. The staff at the facility observed her and let her know when she was behaving seductively with the male patients.

After her discharge, Ava and I began the work of understanding the reasons for each behavior she condemned in herself and finding ways to introduce new behaviors to increase her self-esteem. With the use of tutors, she enrolled in computer classes and business school, a signal to her mother that she deserved her mother's respect. She seemed to be using her mother's value system as a compass to get her bearings, having missed the opportunity to develop self-esteem as a young girl. Her abuse by her father had undermined that development. She would have a difficult time proving to *herself* that she was adequate without first becoming acceptable to her mother. Though working to earn her mother's approval might not seem a reasonable goal of therapy, it was a necessary first step.

Her mother's sudden divorce from her father had helped Ava to view the sexual abuse differently, helping her rid herself of self-blame. It was an expedient development, however, one that is unavailable to most patients.

The next step in therapy would be to revise Ava's choice of men and the masochistic and self-abusive elements of her attraction to, and arousal by, cruel men. Ava had a few "slips" along the way, including occasional cocaine use and flirtation with harmful men, but these episodes were short-lived and eventually disappeared. As of this writing, Ava has been in treatment for four years and probably will need several more years to compensate for the damage done to her during her formative years.

Like Audrey, Ava's recovery from the sexual abuse inflicted by her father was complicated by drug use. One study, in the journal *Addiction*, notes "that survivors reported cocaine . . . as their serious problem drug more frequently than other women. . . ."[6] Certainly drugs and alcohol are widely used as emotional painkillers; teens and adult women who have been abused are vulnerable to addiction. Patients and therapists alike should be aware that addictions form a barrier to successful therapy by diluting the intensity of the therapeutic experience. Therefore, when substance addictions are present, they must be addressed in treatment before meaningful therapy can begin.

15

Maureen:
"Dissociation Just Happens"

Maureen came to therapy for treatment of bulimia. She was thirty-one years old, athletically built, and had an attractive face partially obscured by significant swelling along both jawbones. This reaction is an autoimmune response: the body interprets the constant vomiting as a symptom of infection, so it stimulates glands in the jaw area to secrete fluids to help fight the imaginary infection. The result is this face-distorting swelling.

In addition to being bulimic, Maureen also cut herself.

Maureen had grown up in an unstable family situation. Her parents, both alcoholics, had split up when she was seven and thereafter she took turns living with each of them. By the time Maureen was twelve, her father had been divorced twice and was married for the third time. She learned to keep to herself and tried to avoid "making trouble" for her parents by expressing her feelings or asking for help. When she started to develop physically, her twenty-year-old stepbrother raped her during a time when she was living in her father's blended family. He was too smitten with his third wife to pay attention to her timid allegations, so she ran away to live with her unmarried alcoholic mother. After several months of discord and neglect she returned to her father's house.

The local high school was a mixture of upscale students and a group of toughs from the rundown part of town, which surrounded the factories on the original site of the old city. She didn't fit in with either group at school and had no close friends. She was deathly afraid of her stepbrother and had no one to turn to.

Hoping to enhance her own ability to defend herself, she enrolled in a women's martial arts self-defense course. She eagerly applied herself in the martial arts course and stayed in the program to its top level. To augment her martial arts techniques, she also took up weightlifting. None of this arming of herself calmed her fears of future attacks, though she was confident she would use her strength and skills if ever attacked again. Her stepbrother became aware of her prowess in martial arts and did not attack her again. However, he and his friends occasionally teased her by raising their flexed arms when she walked by. "Hi, Butch!" they would shout in a mock-friendly tone. Their behavior was a constant reminder of the past, and though she sneered at their remarks she occasionally experienced flashbacks to the rape.

After graduating from high school she joined her city's police force. There she was subjected to sexist wisecracks, which she returned with such stinging retorts that the adversaries quickly suggested a truce. This did not give her peace of mind, however. It only perpetuated her perception of being surrounded by men who would assault her or rape her if they could. After leaving the police force she supported herself during the day as an emergency medical technician while attending college at night, graduating in six years, at the age of twenty-five. Men rarely bothered her and when they saw her style of response, they backed off. Despite her childhood rape, she had two romantic involvements with men. Both had ended before she entered therapy during her last year of school.

During her first session with me, her demeanor was subdued, but her defiance and suspicion were unmistakable. She recited the summary of her abuse with her jaw set, as if the events did not matter to her. This mechanical delivery is a defense mechanism often used by victims of sexual assault when reporting the details to the police. Describing these embarrassing details to strangers feels like reliving the original events and inviting others to watch. Distancing themselves emotionally from the events, as if they were talking about someone else, makes the telling more bearable.

After Maureen had given me her history with almost no prompting, I asked her if she saw any connection between her bulimia and the sexual assault by her stepbrother. In a cynical tone, she responded "Not really. Bulimia has helped me tolerate a tough test or paper at school, a bad accident where people were mangled, a teacher who's a pain in the ass, or I guess just about anything. I didn't have bulimia way back when I had trouble with the stepbrother."

"But now it helps you manage the rough spots."

"Yeah, you could say that."

"You know that it's waiting for you at the end of the day like a 'fix,' and that makes the day bearable?"

"You know us junkies—we can tolerate a lot if we know our fix is waiting for us."

"Do things happen that make you anxious during the day, even frighten you?"

"Sure."

"What happens to you when you're frightened?"

"I dissociate. I go away . . . from me. Otherwise I have flashbacks and I have to relive all that old crap again. Not just my mind but my body too. I sweat, my heart pounds, I shake hoping nobody notices. Sometimes it feels like I'm being penetrated, I contract until it hurts or my breasts burn like I was getting groped. Sometimes I go limp because I'm sure I can't stop anything from happening to me, like getting killed."

"This all happens to you at work?"

"It can happen at work, or it can happen anywhere even if nothing is happening."

"So you often don't know when or why it happens?"

"But I know I'll have my bulimia at the end of the day."

"What you're describing is post-traumatic stress. That means anything upsetting can cause you to dissociate."

"No, not necessarily . . . [dissociation] just happens."

"Do you see it diminishing with time?"

"I can never measure that. I don't keep a score sheet. I just don't know. Maybe it'll go away tomorrow, but even then it would take years for me to believe it was really gone. Or maybe it'll be around forever."

"So the flashback trauma can happen without warning?"

"It can."

About a month later I mentioned a behavior of Maureen's to her. "I've noticed that sometimes after a session you write me a stinging note referring to something I said, omitted to say, questioned you about, or said in the wrong way."

"Yeah, sometimes it feels like you blew it, and I wonder why I'm making the sacrifices I do to come here."

"So after we've discussed these incidents and resolved them, do your feelings about them change?" Maureen shrugged her shoulders and gave me a tight-lipped nod. "It seems like a minor misunderstanding turns into reason enough to end your therapy?"

"I guess so."

"So the same way a harmless event can escalate into traumatic proportions and cause you to dissociate, cut yourself, or have a bulimic episode, a statement or comment from me can temporarily cause you to want to cut off therapy, forgetting the entire history of our work together?"

"Yup, that's what it's like to be me."

"I think if we can revise the way you relate to me here in therapy, you'll be able to revise the way you relate to other people and most importantly to yourself."

"Okay, but how do we start that?"

"I guess we are going to try to get you to voice your objection to what I say or how I interpret you at the time it happens, so that it doesn't have time to build up into an extreme reaction which causes you anger, fear, and pain."

Maureen had worked so hard to arm herself against attack that she found it difficult to drop her guard during therapy. When she did, she experienced a need to pull back and rearm with anger. She directed her anger at me because I was the one encouraging her to disclose her feelings. Our first important goal in therapy was to have her reconnect with her feelings and learn to express them without regret.

Fortunately Maureen's motivation to be healthy, despite her fear of living without bulimia, was strong enough for her to begin the difficult work of emotional revision. As of this writing, she is still in therapy to accomplish this.

16

Kendra:
"So I Have to Be *Normal*?"

Kendra was referred to me as an eighteen-year-old with an eating disorder. She had a history of cycling between compulsive overeating (and its accompanying weight gain) and anorexia nervosa. She arrived for our first session well dressed, attractive, and confident. Kendra's comfortable manner was in sharp contrast to that of Deirdre (Chapter 3) or June (Chapter 4), who were shy and timid. Kendra told me about her eating cycles while making strong, seductive eye contact; she assumed provocative postures on the couch.

When she stopped her narrative, indicating that this was the summary of her problems, I asked her if she had ever been sexually abused.

"Yes."

"Was it a family member?" She nodded. "Was it your brother?"

"Well, they were like *brothers*," she responded, emphasizing the plural, "but no, they were actually my cousins. They lived in our two-family home when I was growing up. But they spent all their time with us after their mom was killed in a traffic accident." As she spoke, she retained her composure.

"You don't show signs that it was terrifying or even intimidating."

"I didn't even know it was wrong . . . until I told my friends in the fifth grade, and their parents wouldn't let them play with me anymore. I thought everyone did it."

"Did you regard your cousins' behavior as acceptable or fun?"

"Not so much with my older cousin. He could be mean, but I wasn't really scared of him. At some point he brought my younger cousin into the game. He is a timid personality so I never felt threatened. I have to admit it was pleasurable with both of them. As I said before, I didn't even know it was wrong until other people, including my family, told me. I quit when my older cousin demanded to have sex with me. I still get along with my younger cousin, but I dislike my older cousin—he's generally a bastard."

"Do you think the sex play with your cousins has had any effect on you?"

"Well, I think I'm freer than most girls about sex," she responded glibly.

There was something contradictory about her: despite her presentation as a free and easy girl who enjoyed her sexuality, she had experienced early social stigma and rejection and was suffering with an eating disorder. Her seductive behavior in my office had been a clue to sexual abuse, but in that first session she apparently needed to hold on to the self-image of a girl who felt that sex was fun.

In later sessions Kendra would admit that because she felt like a sexual victim, she usually wanted to be the sexual predator. She described a typical incident in a bar where she opened her blouse and requested a free beer of the male bartender. He stared at her chest for a moment and exclaimed, "Sure!" and brought her the beer. She also talked about insisting on having sex with boys on the first date. We discussed how this was "turning the tables" on the boys and making them the complicit victims.

Kendra then described her pattern of shifting between anorexia and bulimic overeating, as well as the depression that stayed with her most of the time. She was puzzled at these mood and disorder shifts, unable to attribute them to specific events or causes. We discussed the possibility that her worst moments with her cousins never really left her, causing her to behave in ways that denied and overshadowed their persistent presence in her subconscious. During these discussions vivid and explicit memories became conscious for her. We had to reframe her original childhood feelings of self-blame so that she could see herself, as a child, the actual victim of sexual abuse, even though she tried to "make the best of it" by allowing herself to become aroused, even instigating sexual activity herself after it had been going on for a long time.

We spoke about her childhood sense that this was going to continue forever and how she had needed to adjust to it. The side effect of this adaptation was that she learned to see herself as a coconspirator in sexual acts that she later discovered were seen as immoral. She came to think of herself as a bad person, destined to remain so, and needed to feel sexual control as well. Her behaviors increasingly conformed to this idea, creating a consistency that was more comfortable and emotionally tolerable than any attempt to change what she perceived as inevitable.

Kendra paid social penalties for her behaviors. At college, as in high school and grade school, girls would not befriend her since they considered her a whore who might seduce the boy they were involved with. She accepted this and spoke about not liking other girls or wanting their friendship, saying she preferred boys as friends anyway. She chose to deny seeing herself as socially isolated from the college community of girls. The attacks of depression, alternating with bingeing or starving recurred cyclically. She selected boys who were interested in shallow relationships. They were mildly abusive—mostly "one-night stands" who ignored her after an episode of sex. Boys she considered nice or more serious in their desire for a relationship "just don't interest me or turn me on." Occasionally she would lament, "I wish they would."

Kendra was likable and bright; she attended a highly competitive college and was attractive. But none of this helped her feel good about herself. Self-hatred, self-deprecation, and the feeling that she was not fit to belong among her peers dominated her negative self-image. She really did not know how to belong, not since she had been exiled by her peers in the fifth grade. "How many nice girls would befriend a whore?" she protested in one session.

For Kendra, treatment would focus on shedding self-blame for her sexual past, as well as letting go of the characteristic behaviors she had evolved to deal with her negative identity. This process would take time and patience. As she became more aware of her impulses and their causes, she would be able to stop acting on them some of the time. Then they would gradually diminish. She might retain some of her desires for past pleasures, and her sexual impulses might still cause her to view herself negatively, but to a much lesser degree.

"I feel like I'm supposed to start my life all over—but I don't know how."

"You could live a more discreet life, feeling increasingly better about yourself without needing to feel that your childhood experiences never happened."

"So I'll never be 'purified'?"

"If you mean will you feel as if none of this ever happened, and you will never have the slightest impulse in those directions, no."

"So where do we go from here?"

"We try to make the connections between those feelings about yourself and your depression, which we might think of as 'bad ideas about yourself.' We should do the same for your eating-disorder impulses and behaviors. You should always appreciate that they are lurking below the surface waiting to undermine you. We will have to work on getting you to forgive yourself . . . and maybe becoming mad at your cousins for having pleasure at your expense."

"Maybe they had pleasure at my expense, but I also developed a sense of power that most people never experience. What you're asking me to learn is how to give up my power. That's like asking someone who has been a teen television star to be a regular person again, to give up being rich and famous, and go to work at a job that offers her none of the special attention and money that became normal to her. That's not 'normal'—that's oblivion, that's being no one after being someone."

"You're saying that it's a demotion to belong in the mainstream with other young women?"

"Well that's how it feels. You're asking me to join the amateurs after I've been in the big leagues. Maybe being a loner—shunned by other girls and not giving a damn—seems more moral to you than my aggressive sexuality, but that's what keeps me on top of the game."

"Do you think that you'll still feel this way when school is over and you're just another one-night stand to a bunch of nameless, faceless strangers that think of you as an unimportant, unmemorable sexual encounter? They won't be eager, excited, or grateful young college guys, but working men and businessmen maybe twenty or thirty years older than you, and you'll just be the entertainment for the evening."

"That makes me sound like a whore."

"I don't think what you're doing is healthy or good for your self-image."

"So I should give up my edge over the other girls?"

"Yes."

"So I have to become *normal*?"

"You don't have to become *invisible*. You will still be an attractive woman, but you could also go after other areas of achievement that have little to do with appearance."

"What if I'm not good at anything else?"

"You're a smart young woman who's graduating from a competitive college. You'll have to stop coasting on your sexuality and try to succeed in something that takes effort and isn't merely a symptom of how your cousins trained you, something that won't come with depression and bulimia."

"And you think I could succeed?"

"You're asking me that because you don't believe in yourself. Under your sexual bravado, coping with abuse by being seductive has lowered your self-esteem."

"I'm going to miss how easy it is, I guess."

"There'll be more substantial rewards."

Kendra's face seemed to soften into a different kind of smile, one that made her look a little younger. "I hope you're right."

—

Kendra's case demonstrates how a defensive posture, such as sexual aggression, can develop as a result of childhood sexual abuse. The sexual pleasure she experienced with her cousins caused her great internal conflict. To defend against that conflict, she maintained her heterosexuality but kept herself in charge of her sexual activity with men. She often pushed them further than they wanted to go. She was always the initiator and rarely became aroused during these acts; not feeling arousal reassured her that she was in control so that she would never be a sexual victim again.

Kendra's major issue centered on her lack of trust; she needed to be in control in every sexual situation. She compensated for the absence of emotional closeness with aggressive seductiveness. Being in charge sexually helped her to feel safe. But she had buried her sadness and low self-esteem in eating disorders and underlying depression. She was scared to face the world without the edge of flashy sexuality, afraid she could not succeed without it. Owning her real feelings, which had been repressed for so long, would give her the personal power to be herself, to build friendships, and to choose real goals for her future.

An issue that caused Kendra difficulty in treatment was her compulsive need to act glibly and show confidence where she had none, which came off as bravado. In demonstrations of independence, she engaged men in power struggles, including her therapist. It was hard for Kendra to take and use advice, not because she feared betrayal but because she found it hard to believe in anyone. She did not respect men because she could control them with seduction, and she disliked women because they rejected her. During the course of therapy this gradually changed, as she used her newfound trust to form more straightforward relationships with men and began tentative steps toward risking friendships with several women.

Though sexual aggressiveness might not be the expected behavior from an abuse survivor, it is nevertheless an understandable outcome. Recognizing Kendra's sexual behavior as a defensive posture was a key to her treatment.

17

Julie:
Relief from
Psychotic Episodes

Julie was admitted to a psychiatric hospital for bulimia and dissociative disorder, resulting from repeated rapes by her brother's friend when she was twelve years old. She had never disclosed the information about the rapes before. She was nineteen, and this was her fifth hospitalization.

At the time the rapes occurred, she became withdrawn, volatile, and her behavior became erratic. She also developed anorexia and bulimia. These sudden changes puzzled everyone, so she was sent for treatment for what would be the first of several hospitalizations. She was uncooperative during her first four hospitalizations, which occurred over seven years; she did not improve during this time.

Julie was nineteen when she read one of my books on anorexia (*Treating and Overcoming Anorexia*) and sought my help. After consulting with me, she and I decided that she would stay in the Northeast for her fifth hospitalization; she was too emaciated for outpatient treatment in my office, so I would treat her as an inpatient. At the hospital, her initial admission interview was not promising. She stared away from the interviewer and looked out the window for nearly half an hour, saying nothing in response to his questions. He reminded her that she had requested this admission and would be sent home if she could not cooperate during the admission process. Nevertheless, she was admitted. In the hospital treatment program her behavior was passive and though pleasant she volunteered little information about herself. She was not able to initiate conversations. She participated in group therapy and other activities, but only on the periphery.

One day in an individual psychotherapy session we were talking about what I thought would be a nonthreatening subject: I asked her how long she had been bulimic. She leaned forward and tilted to one side, then suddenly thrust her head back, hitting the wall behind her chair with deliberate force. She then brought her head and neck to the same pre-thrusting position, as if preparing to repeat this head-banging maneuver again. I had just enough time to grab the chair's arm support (luckily it was a swivel chair on caster wheels) and pull it away from the wall so that when she thrust her head back a second time, it did not make contact with the wall. The wall was cinder block, and she could have cracked her skull.

She then began to flail about. While restraining her with one arm I was able to call the emergency phone number for nursing assistance. Six nurses came down and immediately sedated her with a hypodermic needle. Three days later, during our next session, Julie protested my having had her sedated and carted off to a seclusion room. I explained to her that when she dissociated in a potentially dangerous way, she had in effect "left the session," leaving in her place an oblivious, thrashing body that needed sedation and restraints. Julie accepted responsibility for provoking my reaction to her behavior, and the therapeutic relationship remained intact.

After several sessions and a second incident of attempted head banging, I asked Julie if she had ever been molested or raped. She started to stare off into space, but I interrupted her to stop her from dissociating. It was apparent that she had memories she needed to cope with. I repeated the question in a gentle but insistent tone.

She came out of her dissociation, turned to me, and began to cry. "Yes, but I don't want to talk about this with you. Can I talk to a woman therapist?"

I assured Julie that we could arrange that with hospital staff. The following day Sylvia, a senior psychologist in the unit, took over the individual therapy.

At the next team meeting Sylvia prepared the members to work with Julie effectively and sensitively by quoting to the staff Julie's account of her history: "It was my brother's friend. He would make me undress and put my knees up to my chest with my arms wrapped around them and then suddenly and violently rape me. I felt crazy while this was going on. It felt like an electric shock in my brain. I wasn't so aware of what was happening as I was about feeling like my brain would explode from it. My brain didn't work for hours afterward. I just couldn't think. I don't even know what happened or what I did during those hours. Now that happens to me randomly. It can happen any time. I was hoping it would get better, but I think it's getting worse."

Julie remained at the hospital for a year, gradually discussing the abuse in individual and group therapy. Her violence and withdrawn behavior diminished markedly. She made a few friends and became more social. About six months later she was discharged to a residential treatment center in her home state. She then moved in with her parents and worked in her community. We talked over the telephone occasionally for several years.

The hospital provided a safe atmosphere where Julie could disclose her abuse, even though the disclosure provoked endangering behavior and psychotic episodes. The therapeutic relationship not only survived these difficulties, but assisted Julie in confronting her abuse.

Julie's story provides us with an example wherein the therapist had to restrain the patient physically and have her chemically sedated while she was an inpatient, without losing her trust and the therapeutic alliance.

18

Doreen: Compulsive Scratching *Is* Self-Mutilation

Doreen was a pleasant-looking girl in her late twenties; she was living with her parents and brother because she was unemployed. She came for treatment of self-mutilation: she was compulsively scratching the skin on her arms, chest, and face. In our first session she spoke apologetically, both about her face, which was streaked with broad red and pink lines, and about being unworthy of help. She cried often. She made angry statements alternately directed toward her family and toward herself. Thus her anger was simultaneously directed inward and outward.

Initially, she spoke about her inability to say no to people who exploited her; this included her boyfriend, who beat her. In later sessions she talked about certain painful childhood experiences. Beginning when she was nine, her fourteen-year-old brother would touch and penetrate her in front others, mocking her at the same time. He would begin by saying things like "Want to see my sister's pussy?" to three or four of his friends who were in the room. Then, without waiting for his audience of curious boys to reply, he would pull down her pants while she tried to squirm away from him, protesting his behavior. It was clear to her that she was his property to show off to his friends.

Unlike even younger children who have been victimized by childhood sexual abuse, Doreen was old enough to experience the full force of embarrassment and humiliation her brother was subjecting her to. When she complained to her parents about him, they would scold him and tell him not to do that sort of thing again. Both parents worked during the day. Perhaps for this reason he was confidently able to ignore their scolding. Eventually Doreen's parents got tired of her complaints, ignoring them instead of taking action against her brother. She recalls her father's annoyance with her when he said in response to her mounting complaints, "Why don't you stop him? Smack him or something!"

Like a younger child, she understood that there was no protection available to her.

Scratching or "picking" at one's skin does not fit into the category of activities therapists normally think of as comprising self-mutilation, but I get many inquiries from individuals wanting to know whether picking or scratching the skin is a form of self-mutilation. It is. Picking and scratching, though lacking the element of endangerment that comes from using a knife, razor blade, or match, nevertheless shares many of the same elements as cutting and burning. These include causing pain (sometimes more pain than cutting) and visible damage, often bleeding and sometimes scarring. Like other forms of self-mutilation, scratching and picking have many causes, and satisfy the same needs: releasing anger toward others or toward oneself through the absorption and distraction of the activity. The pain derived from scratching or picking takes the place of self-punishment or aggression stemming from feelings of victimization, self-loathing, or resentment. In many cases this practice is caused by childhood sexual abuse. Scratching seems less dramatic than cutting or burning, but scratchers and pickers often feel more shame about their behavior than cutters do. Despite its lack of drama, scratching does produce a repulsive appearance and may cause more disapproval by others than cutting does. It therefore can serve as a useful symbolic redress of grievances for the experience of childhood sexual abuse.

In Doreen's case there was the additional factor of embarrassment; by the age of nine she had developed modesty, usually not found in younger children. The reenforcement of the older boys' attention coupled with her parents' reluctance to take serious steps to stop the behavior may have caused Doreen to infer that her victimization was socially acceptable. As we will see, this in turn may have caused her to fuse sexual arousal with pain and embarrassment, resulting in sexual masochism.

Doreen presented herself in therapy as timid, sad, and faintly angry. Her frequent crying was not self-pity but a desperate request for help: she was almost begging for protection. Coupled with her crying was a posture of overly compliant and approval-seeking behavior. Doreen's demeanor could easily produce in others, including a therapist, a desire to protect her. But any would-be helper might become frustrated by her continual abuse of her skin. This could have been part of the initial phase of the therapy process, since all patients test to see whether their therapists will reject them. Any therapist beginning treatment feeling intense pity for the patient runs the risk of becoming frustrated when his or her excessive warmth (an expression of pity) fails to stop the patient from scratching. She could then perceive the therapist's frustration as annoyance at her, which would confirm her feelings of abandonment and self-loathing.

Doreen's feelings about herself had already produced in her another, more dangerous symptom. Her sexual dysfunction expressed itself as *masochism*, the desire to be hurt, humiliated, and dominated by one's sexual partners. Moreover, the intensity of her masochism was escalating. It evolved from slapping, to spanking, to being whipped by a belt on the back of her thighs until she bled. She herself was encouraging her partner to develop an even larger appetite for his sadistic impulses until she was approaching the point where she risked being seriously injured, or even killed.

Doreen often came late to her appointments. This behavior was not only another way for her to experience self-deprivation. It was also a form of *passive aggression* deprivation. One day I asked what Doreen was doing prior to leaving for appointments that would cause her lateness.

She answered, "I was scratching myself, and I thought I could stop on time but I couldn't."

"Did someone hurt or offend you, or did something upsetting happen which caused your inability to stop scratching?"

"No, it's more complicated than that." She sounded shy and ashamed. "I get pleasure from it and didn't want the pleasure to stop."

"Are you saying that you get sexually aroused scratching yourself, that this is a form of masturbation?"

"Yes."

"Then this behavior, like the beatings, is fused with arousal?"

A very shy and ashamed Doreen answered, "Yes."

Several weeks later Doreen surprised me with a change of demeanor. She began the session by energetically protesting about something that had taken place at home. "My brother's sexual assaults on me may be gone, but nothing else has changed. We were walking by each other in the kitchen last week when we brushed shoulders. The second time, we bumped into each other harder. My brother reached down and grabbed my ankle. He pulled me high off the hard kitchen floor and dropped me! The top of my head hit the floor first. . . . I was in blinding pain, not just in my head and neck, but I got ringing in my ears and blurred vision that lasted two days. I was really scared that he had damaged my hearing and my eyesight.

"My parents acted kind for several days, but they didn't take me to a hospital or even a doctor. Instead they tried to minimize what he did to me. I was so unaccustomed to their behaving nicely to me, I think I got confused. Ever since I moved back in the house, they have been complaining. They say they didn't ask me to return home, and they say things like 'Nobody wants you here.' It's really horrible—they just make me feel like dirt. So I settled for the 'gift' of not being picked on, but that came with requests [from them] that I not press charges against my brother. No one seemed to mention the possibility that I might have a concussion, a fractured skull, or bleeding in my brain. Nothing has changed except *where* he's assaulting me! And my parents still won't protect me. In my mind the whole thing connects to the original abuse. . . . it's all the same!"

When Doreen's lateness (due to her compulsive scratching) significantly shortened her sessions to twenty minutes, I took the unusual step of telephoning her at the time she should leave home to get to her session on time. When she answered the phone I said, "It's time to stop scratching and leave for the office." Doreen, apparently relieved by my directiveness and instructions, stopped scratching herself and left for her session. It was a beginning, but we had a great deal of therapeutic work ahead. This would include reshaping her feelings about her femininity and repairing her masochistic sexuality, which was a direct result of her childhood sexual abuse.

For Doreen, her legacy from childhood sexual abuse became not only her choice of men who related nastily toward her, but the self-harming and sometimes self-mutilating behaviors she learned to require as sexual stimulation. Repairing the psychological damage Doreen sustained in childhood, especially in light of the unchanged family situation, was to be a major undertaking. The first step was to encourage and guide her toward taking advantage of the help that was available to her in therapy.

19

Jen:
A Case of Iatrogenic Abuse

The preceding chapters in Part Two present case histories of childhood sexual abuse that, though varied, all feature a perpetrator and his victim. Jen's story illustrates a somewhat atypical case in that she experienced violation that was emotionally and physically akin to sexual abuse. She was repeatedly forced to endure a medical procedure that centered on her urogenital area. However, the resulting trauma (pain, penetration, debasement, fear, and helplessness) was unintentional on the part of the physician. Illness, disability, or other forms of harm caused inadvertently by a physician, hospital staff, or medication are called *iatrogenic*.

Jen came into therapy alarmed at her self-mutilating behavior; she was cutting herself with a knife, and she had just read my book on cutting. She was a nineteen-year-old college sophomore, who looked younger than her age, though she was quite pretty and flirtatious. Her parents were divorced, and she lived in a large apartment with her father, who was traveling most of the time. She had an estranged relationship with her mother after living with her for seven years following the divorce. She told her mother that she had fears that her new stepfather was sexually attracted to her, though he never misbehaved toward her. As soon as Jen said this, her mother asked her to leave the house and move in with her father.

She came to treatment a short time later. After several weeks of treatment she displayed other symptoms in addition to the cutting.

For example, one day about this time my phone rang. It was Jen calling from the office where she worked part time as a dental assistant. She sounded desperate. Her voice was loud, intense, shrill, and raspy.

"I can't see! I don't know what I'm doing! I'm unable to work! I'm calling you from the supply closet from my cell phone!"

"Jen, do you mean you're disoriented? Have you been having problems with your vision?"

"You don't understand. I don't know what's going on. The other assistant is trying to keep me calm."

"Are you having a panic attack?"

"I suppose so." She experienced a moment of calm followed by her fright escalating and her voice getting louder again. "I just don't know what's going on!"

"Do you have medication with you?"

"Yes I have that antianxiety stuff Dr. Stern prescribed for me."

"What dosage are you supposed to take?"

"I don't know. It's one pill at a time."

"Call him and ask him if you could take two. I want you to call me back an hour after you've taken the meds. Stay where you are, and tell your boss that you don't feel well and you have to lie down. I'm sure he'll be sympathetic."

She responded with a docile "Okay."

She called back an hour later to say, "I'm still not feeling so good, but I think I can go home by myself."

"Call me when you get home."

Again that childlike, docile "Okay." The phone rang again a half hour later. "It's me. I can't find my building."

"Where are you?"

"On a street corner."

"Is it your street corner?"

"I don't know."

"Read me the signs on the lamppost."

"Oh, yeah, it's my corner."

"Turn around in the direction of your building and start walking toward it."

"Okay."

"Do you see the front entrance yet? Do you see the doorman?"

"Yes, yes! I'm almost there!"

"Good. Now go upstairs and take a shower or bath and call me when you're finished."

An hour later she was calmer, but she had cut herself in the shower. We both agreed that the cut did not sound serious. Jen had no idea where her father was, nor did she know when he would return to the apartment. She thought it might be a day or two. She agreed to go to bed.

The next day she came for a session, and we talked about the episode the night before.

"I have other things that happen to me. I lose time. I mean, I look at my watch and three hours have gone by, and I have no idea where I've been or what I've done. Sometimes I only lose minutes, or even seconds. I crashed my father's car into a tree while I was out of it. I guess you could call it a trance or something, but I still don't remember what happened. I never do."

"Does any event or person ever provoke these trances or, to be more clinical, dissociative episodes?"

"No. It's like I just go away, but to nowhere."

"When was the first time this ever happened to you?"

She thought for a minute. "In the hospital: I was seven years old and I had a condition called 'urinary reflux,' which meant that my urine was backing up from my bladder to my kidneys. There's an operation for that, but my urologist thought it would be better if he could teach me how to urinate correctly so it wouldn't back up and endanger my kidneys. They put me on this table and put this catheter into my urethra, which hurt plenty, not to mention that I was embarrassed to death. I was a seven-year-old girl naked, since they pulled the gown up, with several men aside from my doctor who were in the room. You know, sometimes I think they were enjoying watching."

"Was this a onetime procedure?"

"Oh no," she laughed a sardonic laugh. "It went on once or twice a month for four years. I would beg my mother the night before each time not to take me there, but she would explain that it was for my health and the doctor felt it was necessary. I would cry all night but I had to go the next morning anyway. Sometimes my father would take me. One of them [my parents] was always present in the room. I remember my father saying to me repeatedly while they were pumping this fluid into my bladder, 'It's medical, Jen.' And when they finished pumping the fluid in, they had a meter that registered how evenly I was peeing, and if it varied too much they would do it again. So I had to concentrate as hard as I could to release my bladder as evenly as possible, to avoid the torture being repeated. When I finished, I had peed all over myself on the table. It was so embarrassing with all those men watching. I learned to 'go away' and leave my body behind. I guess I still did the 'correct' behavior, but I learned to stop feeling that I was there so it would be bearable.

"This went on for four years and it failed. I still had urinary reflux, so they did the operation anyway. I guess it was for nothing. Then, after the operation, I thought I finally had it beat, that it was over. I was told I had to go back to that horrible room for them to do the same test to make sure the operation was a success. I didn't want to go back because I was eleven and I was beginning to grow pubic hair and I didn't want them to see that. To this day I still can't stand it when a guy I'm with wants to see my vagina or go down on me. Last week I was in school and the art teacher showed Picasso's *The Prostitutes*. I lost it and started screaming at him. He and the rest of the class thought I was crazy. They kept asking me, 'Are you all right?' I guess I seemed pretty crazy to them, and I guess I was at the time. My visual memories of those medical procedures were my thighs, knees in the air and spread apart. Picasso's painting had such a similar perspective of the prostitutes' thighs, it just took me back to that room. I felt like I was really back there."

Jen's experiences contained all the elements of sexual abuse from her point of view: she was forced to submit to painful penetration in a sexual area repeatedly over a period of four years. She had no way to escape and no protectors: her parents, who were present, instructed her to submit. She was undressed, which was humiliating. And the experience was perceived as unendingly repetitive (again, prompting her to feel the "forever factor"). That the physician was unaware of the future psychological damage he was doing, merely viewing this procedure from a medical standpoint, is a problem that often arises in pediatric urology and gynecology, and with pediatric gastroenterology when it deals with the rectal area. Despite the absence of intentional abuse, the *experience* of sexual abuse occurs with the accompanying serious post-traumatic stress disorder. In Jen's case the physician and everyone else present in the room did a poor job of understanding the emotional impact of their procedures on a young girl. There was no attempt at discretion or pain control, or to listen to the child's objections and feelings.

Medical specialists should evaluate the need for such procedures. When they are unavoidable, then it becomes essential to develop interpersonal sensitivity in this extraordinarily delicate doctor-patient relationship, and to administer the necessary medication or anesthesia to reduce or eliminate pain. Doing so will help avoid causing the serious, sometimes lifelong psychological damage that can result when specialists view these events as simple medical procedures.

During her second year of psychotherapy, Jen went through a period during which she experienced frequent psychotic episodes. One day she came to a session wearing a new hat, jacket, gloves, and skirt. The store tags (consisting of price tags and strings) were hanging from each garment. I inquired whether she was aware of the tags.

She smiled, responding that she liked them and had no intention of ever taking them off.

Jen had apparently done a lot of shopping recently, because for several sessions thereafter she came in with many store tags dangling from her clothing. After the third session with tags still present on her clothes, I asked Jen why she hadn't removed them.

In a young child's voice and at an abnormally loud volume, Jen replied, "I told you I would never take my tags off. I think they look very good, and there's no reason to remove them."

I asked her if she thought that others agreed with her. She replied, "Well, some people are looking at me funny in the street—but I don't care." In a voice becoming even more childish and louder, she pointed at some of the tags with her index finger as if she were teaching a student a lesson on fashion. "These are the strings and these are the tags. That's how the doctor began each session when he was about to catherize my urethra so he could teach me how to pee. He would touch my genitals with his index finger and say, 'These are the labia and this is the urethra.' "

"Jen, do you think that you're displaying your clothing tags, which are not meant to be displayed, in the same way your doctor 'displayed' your genitals, which embarrassed you? Perhaps you're both protesting the 'display' and proving you can tolerate it to yourself and anybody else who sees them—the tags or your genitals."

"I don't know—I told you I like the tags."

Several weeks went by and Jen continued to wear her clothing tags to therapy. I did not repeat my interpretation of the possible relationship between the tags and the medical procedure. Instead, Jen reintroduced the topic. "I know what you think about my tags—maybe it's true. I know I still hate the doctors." Then she started shouting and crying, "It was always horrible! I tried to get used to it! I tried to be a good patient like my parents told me to! But I could *never* stand it! They kept saying it was 'only medical and necessary.' I hated it all, but . . . who the hell could I turn to, to get me out of this nightmare? Not my parents! It must have been me. I just couldn't accept it! I was weak! I guess other kids or people could accept the treatment, but I couldn't!"

"Jen, maybe you weren't weak. Maybe the situation would be difficult, if not impossible, for any girl your age to tolerate without having to blame herself. Maybe this procedure and the doctor's behavior coupled with your wish to be a good patient made you snap. Maybe you can take your tags off now, and metaphorically 'cover yourself up' and recover your dignity, and accept that you deserve that dignity."

Jen asked me if I had scissors. I gave her a pair, and she cut each tag off. She looked at me through angry, tearful eyes and said. "I'm going home and cutting off all the tags on all my clothing!" After that session all the tags disappeared from her clothing.

Some patients who experienced sexual abuse or similar trauma in childhood have psychotic or dissociative episodes, and chaotic thoughts and feelings as adults. Whether or not these are the presenting problem when they enter therapy, such patients may eventually use the therapeutic relationship to get relief from their symptoms, if they trust the relationship. For example, in her college classroom Jen would have outbursts so severe that other students thought she was crazy. In addition to that social consequence, Jen could become so disoriented that she could not find her way home, even though she was within a city block of her apartment house; she had to call me on her cell phone to get her bearings. Though psychotic behavior was not the reason she had sought therapy, during the course of her treatment she used her contact with me, in or out of the office, to regain her sense of reality. Eventually she was able to incorporate my help so that she could function independently.

Jen's inappropriate behavior became less frequent and less intense. Gradually her mood improved until most of the time she was steady and even-tempered and only occasionally moody. She has applied to graduate school. Though she still has episodes of unreasonable volatility, they are extremely infrequent and short-lived. We will continue to work together until her behavior no longer threatens her social and romantic relationships, school, or work. Jen is also taking medication that regulates her moods and impulsivity, as well as a low dose of an antipsychotic that will limit the frequency, intensity, chaos, and despair caused by these episodes. At some point she will probably discontinue one or both medications as her life and confidence solidify.

PART THREE

■

UNDERSTANDING
STOLEN
TOMORROWS

20

Trauma

To understand the long-lasting effects of childhood sexual abuse, we need to examine how these traumatic events act on the human brain. Trauma overwhelms the brain's organizational system. In childhood sexual abuse the nature of the trauma is determined by distinct factors which we will discuss in this chapter.

THE CHEMICAL AND PHYSICAL EFFECTS OF TRAUMA ON THE BRAIN

Since childhood experiences are the foundation of all subsequent personality development, damage and corruption of that foundation will weaken the structure of that personality as the person grows into adulthood. The child's earliest impressions reside in the *limbic system*, the collective name for structures in the human brain involved in emotion, motivation, and associating emotion with memory. Signals passing through the limbic system are then relayed to other parts of the brain, including the cerebral cortex, where they are interpreted and given meaning. The limbic system thus acts like a colored gel placed in front of a slide projector: all the colors of the picture viewed on the screen (the cortex) are changed after passing through the gel. The picture will be seen differently depending on what color gel was used. The viewers may not even be able to detect the coloration: unless they are savvy about the effect of different gels on the resulting images (are both old enough and practiced in self-reflection to examine feelings and situations objectively), the pictures will seem natural.

So it is with the molested child: as she grows to adulthood, she is continually affected by her earlier victimization, not even aware of how her perspective has been altered. Her adaptations will seem reasonable to her because, like the gel, her unconscious (seated in the limbic system in the brain) cannot be perceived. She is reacting to her discolored screen.

Her brain has been changed because it was altered while still growing. We often speak of someone being "chemically imbalanced." There is a popular misconception that all of these chemical imbalances in the brain are genetic. Not true. Life experiences can change the way the brain functions physically, and these changes, though they can be profound, are not necessarily permanent.

Almost raped: How the effects of trauma can grow A seventeen-year-old patient of mine was successfully fighting off a would-be rapist who had dragged her into the interior of her mini-van. When he heard another man approaching with a large barking dog, the attacker jumped out and ran to his car, which was parked directly in front of her van. The patient leapt forward into the driver's seat of her van and took down his license number before he could drive away. Her attacker was arrested within two hours and brought into custody.

Due to her vehement resistance, he had not had a chance to touch her in any sexual area or tear off her clothing nor had she been physically harmed. She, on the other hand, while fighting him off had been dreading losing that fight, anticipating being raped and killed. Although she was not a young child at the time of attack, she nevertheless experienced all the trauma, desperation, and helplessness felt by a child being sexually assaulted.

She was regarded as a hero in her town and publicized as one, yet her traumatic experience had profoundly changed her sense of personal safety. Within six weeks of the event she began to fear going out of the house. Whenever she did so, she had her mother at her side. If a man walked in her direction, she would cross the street. Her fears of being attacked grew until she rarely left her home. She had nightmares of men pursuing her and frequent panic attacks when alone in a room. She remained in a state of anxiety most of the time.

She had triumphed in avoiding rape, and had helped the police arrest the perpetrator and put him in jail to await trial. One might think she should have experienced this experience as a close call—she had gotten away and gotten justice. Intellectually she knew this, but the amygdala, the part of the brain that records extreme endangerment into memory, does not process events in an orderly perspective the way the hippocampus does, leaving the cortex unable to organize the event. (The hippocampus is a collection of cells in the brain that files away orderly memories.) The amygdala, which stores memories that involve overwhelming events and does not limit memories to time and place, also plays a key role in processing emotions. It both produces and responds to nonverbal signs of anger, fear, and danger. The amygdala can be easily stimulated into such intense feelings that the person feels as if she is reliving and re-creating the worst moments of the stress-inducing event: she is having "a flashback."

If one event, such as this attempted rape, can change the mental and emotional sensitivities of a seventeen-year-old (who has the perspective of a young adult), how much more profoundly might the brain of a young child who has undergone repeated sexual violations—with their accompanying terrors, pain, and "forever factor"—be changed? We cannot measure the changes since childhood in the amygdala of a patient who is now adolescent or adult; we can only infer these changes from observing the patient's behaviors and listening to his or her stories. However, if such measurements were technologically (and ethically) possible, we would be able to appreciate the need to chemically diminish the amygdala's disruptive power.

EXPERIENCING TRAUMA

When childhood sexual abuse results in trauma for the victim, it means that as the child grows, her fear of the event reoccurring does not diminish. Unlike ordinary unpleasant experiences, traumatic experiences bypass the brain's ability to put them in perspective in terms of the length of time the event took place; the specific details of the scenario; her age; and the likelihood of recurrence, damage, or death. In other words, traumatic experiences, unlike ordinary ones, cannot be "placed" in the past. This leaves the victim vulnerable to emotionally reexperiencing the event at any time, sometimes repeatedly over her entire lifetime. When something, someone, or someplace reminds her of the event, both mind and body react as if it were recurring in the present. Her heart rate increases and blood pressure rises; perspiring and trembling may occur. These unconscious reactions are part of the body's *fight-or-flight response,* a holdover from living in the wild, when, like other animals, we needed the ability to overcome sudden physical dangers in order to survive.

In the most severe cases of abuse, the person goes limp, as if in a trance. This last response occurs if the brain believes death is imminent and nothing can be done to prevent it—the fight-or-flight response has been overpowered.

The entire experience, whether relatively mild or severe, is called a *flashback*. Flashbacks themselves may diminish with time, but the fear of having them is difficult to extinguish. The despair over their recurrence is what I call the "forever factor." This pessimism affects personality growth, assertiveness, and ambition. It also diminishes confidence that social and personal relationships might benefit the individual.

CHILDHOOD SEXUAL ABUSE:
UNIQUE AMONG TRAUMAS

What makes sexual violation a different kind of trauma is that it is an intensely personal debasement and demoralization for the victim. This leaves the victim feeling physically corrupt and morally stained. It does not matter how old the victim is, but the younger the victim the more intense the feeling. This is because children have the smallest vocabulary with which to defend themselves, so their responses to trauma consist of only raw feelings. Later (Chapter 29) we will meet Colleen, who is the most extreme example of this, since she was vaginally penetrated by her father when she was approximately one year old. She did not talk yet, but remembers the raw feelings described above, including tactile and visual, and was able for the first time to superimpose words that fit the feelings only at age sixteen.

Older children and adolescents feel shame and humiliation in addition to what younger children feel. Their only compensation is that they can conceptualize the events verbally and with help defend their sense of integrity using a previously developed sense of self.

Trauma can occur in a variety of ways, such as the shock of seeing something tragic occur. After witnessing the collapse of the towers at the World Trade Center on 9/11, many people are being treated for post-traumatic stress disorder, even though they were not physically injured and might have seen this from several miles away. Loss of a loved one, including pets, can have traumatic effects. Automobile accidents, fires, war experiences—all can produce personality-changing trauma and produce a variety of anxiety disorders.

Trauma from childhood sexual abuse has elements rarely seen in other sources of trauma. The most profound sense of violation, as described earlier, involves penetration of the body vaginally, rectally, or orally. The perpetrator is *inside the body* and communicating indifference or pleasure at the helplessness of the victim, often derisively, whether this communication is explicit or implied. After the traumatic event has occurred, the child may perceive anyone as a potential abuser. She may see herself as an object of derision in other relationships. Sexual abuse is always experienced as being interpersonal, affecting all other relationships she may develop. Given this intense connection between violation and perpetrator, treatment has to be based on a corrective relationship that is more lengthy and intense than treatment for trauma—and trauma-based disorders—from other causes.

FACTORS INDUCING TRAUMA

Several factors determine whether or not trauma producing dissociation in the victim occurs during childhood sexual abuse: the formal relationship of the abuser to the abused, the frequency of the abusive events, and characteristics of the abuser's behavior. We will examine all three of these factors in this section.

The formal relationship between abuser and abused   In most cases of childhood sexual abuse, the greatest predictor of personality distortion and emotional destruction is the nature of the relationship between the child and the perpetrator. It will determine her level of fearfulness, as well as her tendency to be confused about the meaning of the events and to blame herself for causing them. It can cause the deepest psychiatric damage, resulting in dissociation.

The "power" of the perpetrator determines the degree of powerlessness the abused person feels. Several aspects contribute to how much power the abuser has in the abusive relationship. One is age. To a child, all adults have natural authority over her, simply because they are older and bigger. Thus an older adult stranger or acquaintance who abuses her has more power than a younger one would. If the adult has obvious status in the community, such as being her clergyman, teacher, or doctor, then the perpetrator gains additional authority—and hence power—in the eyes of the child. When there is a formal relationship between abuser and abused, the "closer" the formal familial tie, the greater the power. For example, a daughter is at an extreme disadvantage against her father; in most cases, he is the ultimate authority figure in her life, and she has very little ability to question his behavior, much less assert herself.

The child's powerlessness to defend herself and express anger at the attacker, or even to attribute responsibility for injuries and pain caused by the assault to her assaulter, leaves her no alternative but to blame herself and to loathe herself for her weaknesses. Moreover, when older authoritative figures (such as uncles, strangers, clergymen, or fathers) sexually exploit children, the victims are left with the "forever factor" (the belief that the assaults will continue permanently), which causes serious psychological disturbances. These include thought disorders, *psychosis* (a break with reality), multiple personality disorder (also known as dissociative identity disorder), dissociation or trancelike states accompanied by amnesia, self-destructive behaviors, and suicide. (We will describe these conditions and disorders in more detail in Chapter 26.) Such severe disturbances can also occur when the perpetrator is not significantly older than the victim or does not have formal authority, but can use his physical strength, his personality, or both to bully her.

The frequency of the events   Generally, the closer the perpetrator is to the abused, the greater the frequency of abuse. When the perpetrator lives with his potential victim, there are usually more opportunities for him to isolate the child than if the abuser is a family member—or "family friend"—who visits the home.

The frequency of abusive events, in turn, affects the nature of the survivor's response to her perpetrator and the severity of the psychological damage she sustains. For example, when an abusing visitor comes infrequently to the house the potential victim has a chance to martial her resources to avoid him, to stay away from home when he is expected, even to hide in the house for the duration of the visit. Adrienne (Chapter 6) as a child spent as much as three hours under her bed whenever her uncle came. Not until after she heard the door slam as he left would she come out, sneezing from the dust. During visits when the whole family headed for the beach, she knew her uncle would seek her out to play "games" with her in the water, and then she would be trapped. But because he lived outside the home and was an infrequent visitor, arriving only two to three times a month, Adrienne had time to think about his acts in between visits and to develop the ability to hate and blame him for the abuse. She did not suffer from the self-loathing or trauma states that a greater frequency would have created.

Rose, on the other hand, was at the mercy of her uncle, who lived in the family home and babysat for her. He raped her frequently, and the blood and pain she vividly remembered caused her to become mentally chaotic, have psychotic episodes, and cut herself frequently. She resorted to magical thinking (imaginary tricks to stop the assaults), which did not work. She experienced panic attacks if she was indoors with any man even when women were present. Because of the frequency of the initial episodes of abuse, she lived in constant fear of future assault by her uncle. Her mind was overwhelmed into trauma states; these were provoked easily, happening more often and lasting longer than if her uncle had been just a visitor.

The abuser's behavior toward his victim   If the abuser is frightening, brutal, verbally nasty and insulting, he will cause nearly all the worst kinds of personality damage mentioned so far: Self-hatred, panic attacks, psychosis, dissociation, perpetuation of abusive behavior, exhibitionism, demand for sexual domination or submission, self-harming behaviors, eating disorders, cutting or other self-mutilation, as well as the harming of others (though the last is less frequent in female than in male survivors).

If instead the abuser is warm, seductive, convincing in his assertion that what he wants to do is not wrong, he might arouse his victim and convince her that they are having fun. This will cause her confusion and may prompt her to seek out this behavior with others. This was the case with Kendra, who learned that she could be sexually powerful with boys and men. Kendra also paid enormous social penalties among girls, and later women, who found her untrustworthy and refused to be friends with her.

In June's case (Chapter 3), her brother would alternate gentle, seductive behavior with violent rape, causing her to fuse romance and sex with abuse. As a result she spent her teens and early twenties involved with boys and men who manifested the same combination of inconsistent qualities in their personalities to which she had become accustomed. Fortunately, June's adaptations did not develop past fear into dissociative trauma, but the formation of her personality was altered. Her choice of behavior within a relationship and of the kind of men she would have relationships with was severely affected. She found herself attracted to abusive men who treated her with indifference or cruelty. The abuse by her brother caused her to make unhealthy choices and, as she put it, to "waste years of my life being attracted to and marrying people who were harmful to me."

In Part IV, we will examine helpful and unhelpful ways to approach and treat survivors of trauma caused by childhood sexual abuse.

21

The Survivor's Relationship
to Her Body

"Sometimes I just want to get crazy glue and glue it shut," stated one discouraged survivor of childhood sexual abuse, referring to her vagina. Survivors rarely feel that the abuse will ever be over, even when it occurred in the distant past. They stay constantly on guard for future possibilities. Women who were abused as children repeatedly apply that "forever factor" every day. In their minds, it is never safe for them to believe that the abuse is over.

During the period when the girl is being abused and before she understands that the abuser is to blame, the only way she can make sense of these terrible events is to relate them to her own body. She decides that they must be provoked by her body, especially those parts of her body that are being assaulted. Part of her attitude is to try not to want to become familiar with these awful places. Often she becomes angry that they exist to tempt her abuser. Many survivors maintain these attitudes throughout their lifetimes but conceal them or their effects from themselves and others. These survivors do not want any stigma from the past to be identified in the present. During episodes of abuse the young child experiences fear, terror, guilt, and pain. As she grows up, she both invents meanings for these experiences and takes in society's meanings for them.

Invented meanings include such internal statements as "I deserve this and must try to stop provoking it." Or "There are parts of my body that make trouble for me. I wish I didn't have them. I hate them and never want to look at them or touch them if I don't have to. I never want anybody else to see those parts of my body either." This latter attitude is not modesty but a fear that if anyone else sees the offending parts of her body, the other person will either be provoked or repelled by them, or will remind her of the assaults.

All young abused girls initially experience terror and pain, and wish to develop strategies to avoid further assault. As the child approaches puberty, the meanings of her assaults evolve as she contends with the physical changes in her body. Her attitudes and feelings may prompt her to intensify her campaign of minimizing her body's sexuality, or she can go to one of two other extremes to gain control: capitalizing on her female sexuality or developing a male image.

MINIMIZING HER FEMALENESS

Puberty brings the sexually abused child a sense of increased danger, which intensifies hatred for her body and can lead to anorexia nervosa and self-mutilation. For the child who was molested before her breasts developed and may still be experiencing abuse, breast development can be frightening: breasts provide a potentially new target for molestation. Diminishing her breasts by losing weight may then seem like a good solution. Extreme weight loss can diminish all signs of maturing femininity, since estrogen production decreases dramatically with weight loss.

As she gets older, modesty, which develops naturally in girls around this time, adds embarrassment and humiliation to the memory and experience of present or past sexual assaults. This intensifies the fear of becoming familiar with her body or knowing anything about her sexual organs. Inquiries into—indeed, any talk about—her feminine development produce anxiety.

PROMOTING HER SEXUALITY

After several childhood years of blaming her body and attempting to minimize her sexual attractiveness, she may develop instead the opposite strategy of promoting her sexuality in order to protect herself. This may seem paradoxical, but the survivor has her own logic. She decides that her most worthwhile aspects are those that were sought after by her abuser. As she matures physically, she attempts to entice other men besides the abuser to seek her out for the same reasons. This suggests that her self-esteem is centered on what she will later call her "sexual desirability" but allows little else. She develops a precocious, flirtatious, or seductive repertoire of behaviors that bring condemnation from girls her age and sexual pursuit from boys her age. She may consolidate her social life along these lines into adulthood, avoiding friendships with girls and seeking attention from boys.

This "solution" to managing the emotional pain of sexual abuse may lead her to make poor choices in boys and men with whom to demonstrate her prowess. Her unconscious need to protect herself by taking control of the sexual situation—control she never had as a child—goes askew, however, as it leads her to choose abusive men, who may beat or even rape her.

In other cases, the desire for control leads her to choose sex-related work: she may become a stripper, to vent her anger at men by ritually teasing them; a prostitute, to make men pay for a sexual experience that means nothing to her; or a porn actress, to verify her degradation. In each of these activities or roles, she is attempting to prove to herself that she does not care about her former abuse, that she can rise above her history, and that by doing so she will be immune to the fear, humiliation, and pain, of both present and past.

IDENTIFYING WITH THE MALE AGGRESSOR

Some adolescent girls and women take on a masculine appearance, gait, speaking style, dress, and facial expression. Having concluded that being and looking female is what made them vulnerable to abuse as children, they become the very image of masculinity so that no predator would consider them a person to assault. They may work out so as to both enhance their masculine appearance and realistically improve their ability to defend themselves.

In Chapter 5 we met Gina, who played the masculine role convincingly in an attempt to deal with the grotesque behaviors she had been subjected to by her father and brothers as a young girl. Nothing short of projecting invincibility through her appearance and forsaking any connection with men socially or sexually could convince her she would remain safe.

An adult who experienced sexual abuse as a child has a complex and difficult relationship with her own body. She has lived with an unspoken question that deeply affects her attitudes toward herself and others: did her body cause the abuse? When her doubt becomes conviction, she may develop extreme behaviors and, in some cases, distrust and even hatred of her physical self. These negative feelings about her female body combine with a child's natural tendency toward self-blame, leading her to expect bad treatment from herself and others. In the next two chapters, we will see how this negative relationship with her body drives her to act out these beliefs.

22

Self-Mutilation

D o abused children grow up with low self-esteem, identity, and femininity problems? They suffer from just about every one of these, including difficulty with trust, attachment, and dependency. In over thirty years of treating patients, I have found that there is a correlation between this disorder and childhood sexual abuse of at least 30 percent.

More than one-third of the self-mutilators—cutters and cutters who sometimes also burn themselves—I have treated were sexually abused or raped in childhood. They were referred to me, or referred themselves, because of the self-mutilation. Most of the mutilation involves cutting. Sometime at the end of the first year of treatment, or earlier if they've been in treatment previously, they volunteer information about the abuse. The relationships between the survivors and their abusers vary widely, as described previously.

Most cutters I have treated (about 90 percent) began hurting themselves sometime between eleven and twenty years of age. The average period of time they have been cutting when discovered by an adult or when they decide on their own to seek treatment is one to two years. This period of hidden cutting has been shortened in recent years due to increased awareness of the phenomenon by professionals and the public.

THE GENERAL PROFILE OF SELF-MUTILATORS

Girls and women who mutilate themselves have difficulty with trusting and depending on others. They generally have low self-esteem, problems with their identity, trouble accepting their femininity, and they suffer from alienation—they feel as if they do not belong to any group or feel close to anyone. They also lack the language for reflecting on their feelings, and generally they do not understand the nature of their emotional pain. They know only that they feel powerless to redress their grievances.

In many cases, self-mutilation is the mind's way of expressing self-blame. The child does not allow herself to blame her parents, fearing their anger or their fragility. Her own negative feelings, such as disappointment in her relationship with her parents, are repressed and turned on herself, because blaming them is unacceptable—they might get angry and reject her for expressing her feelings.

The result is that they experience a verbally undefined pain for which they find a nonverbal solution. As described in Chapter 2, they *reframe* the physical pain into an intense emotional feeling, which feels better than the unexpressed anger, anxiety, or lack of any feeling at all. For cutters especially, their ritual of making small cuts, watching them bleed for a few minutes, and then bandaging themselves provides roughly one to two hours of relaxation. Cutting may begin as a reaction to a random yet serious verbal insult or physical threat and, as time goes on, is used for less serious emotional or social setbacks. Soon they are cutting themselves at any low point in their mood cycle. Eventually they do so just because they have gone "too long" since their last cut, at that point cutting has become an addiction.

Burning is more painful than cutting. It is used to relieve the most intense emotional pain when cutting fails.

TYPES OF CUTTERS

Most cutters fall into one of several categories. Angry cutters are usually people who cannot or are afraid to express discomfort, anger, or rage toward another individual with whom they have grievances. As one patient said to me on her first interview, "I cut myself so I don't cut anyone else." This does not seem quite so strange after considering how commonplace it is for "normal" people to express frustration or anger about another person who is not present by mildly hurting themselves. For example, someone might pound one fist with the other until it hurts, so that the pain becomes a substitute gratification for what might have been an interpersonal confrontation. Banging one's head against a wall or punching oneself, usually on the head, might be done for the same reasons. The angry cutter is more aware of the source of her anger but is incapable of expressing it, either because she anticipates there will be negative consequences (to her job, a relationship, or her social standing) or because she has difficulty being assertive.

Angry cutters are psychologically the "healthiest" group of cutters and have more awareness and a better sense of mental organization than other types of cutters.

Depressed cutters are more random and less predictable in their behaviors. The cutting episodes may be more frequent and the reasons for an episode harder to determine. Medication must be employed to treat the depression and to determine its origins. Chronic or long-term cutting associated with depression usually becomes addictive. The depressed cutter may also be a survivor of childhood sexual abuse.

Dissociative cutters are the most endangered cutters psychologically. These people go into a trancelike state before cutting, and have little or no control over the depth or length of the cut. A psychologist I was treating for cutting often dissociated. One day before driving off to work, she dissociated, took out her knife, made a deep cut on her inner thigh, and put the knife away. Only as she was starting the car did she notice the stream of blood running down her leg. She promptly drove herself to the nearest emergency room for eighteen stitches. She had a history of being repeatedly sexually molested by her brother as a child.

The most difficult self-mutilators to treat are those who dissociate because they are most likely to have experienced some sort of trauma in childhood, often sexual abuse. If that abuse came from within the family, the emotional damage is deeper and becomes much more difficult to bring out and treat.

The next section examines disorders that sometimes result from sexual trauma.

TREATMENT FOR SELF-MUTILATION

In the same way that the presenting problem of anorexia has to be treated before therapy to recover from the underlying emotional causes can begin, especially because of the physical danger, self-mutilation also has to be addressed in the early stages of treatment. Treatment for cutters nearly always requires the use of medication.

Psychotherapy for self-mutilators   Therapists who treat people who cut or burn themselves must be comfortable with seeing blood and skin injuries. Since this is the nature of the way the patient seeks relief, it must be viewed as such; a frightened or angry reaction from the therapist will end treatment right then and there. Therapists can further protect themselves from nonproductive reactions by establishing an outpatient support team. This could include a dermatologist for cuts that need examining and a plastic surgeon for repair of severe cuts and burns. If the therapist is a nonmedical professional, then the team should also include a psychopharmacologist, to make a psychiatric assessment and prescribe medication. The therapist's willingness to get involved with the patient's professional care, especially by setting up such a treatment team, sends a message to a patient that counteracts her pessimistic ideas that no one can help her. This treatment is "good intimate care" as opposed to "bad intimate harm."

Therapy develops the trust that enables a patient to risk experiencing and expressing what to her are vague but intense feelings. Using another person to help her, she can negotiate this difficult process of revealing, clarifying, and revising them. These intense feelings likely include mistrust of her parents and at the same time a fear of betraying the family and guilt at "telling on" her parents. And no matter how much hostility she may feel toward them, she also is anxious about separating from them and afraid of being rejected or abandoned by them. These anxieties create conflict. In fact, many patients find it possible after some psychotherapy to examine the family relationship successfully, disclosing the abuse in family sessions, confronting the abuser if need by, and sharing her real feelings. In addition, in the process of examining her worry about and anger toward her parents her realization and expression of anger or disappointment emerges. This allows her to revise these feelings enough so that, over time, she can let go of her "need" for self-mutilation.

Some therapists refer to the therapeutic process as a "reparenting experience" for the patient. If she has severely conflicted feelings about one or both parents, the therapist might be wise to stay away from that comparison. Clearly the first and most important task for the therapist is to establish trust, safety, and confidence, which can be achieved by displaying, in a sensitive fashion, whatever knowledge and understanding the therapist possesses about self-mutilation.

Treating self-mutilators with accompanying disorders   In addition to self-mutilators who suffer from anger, depression, and dissociative disorders, there are self-mutilators who are diagnosed with one or more other disorders. These include (but are not limited to) generalized anxiety disorder, bipolar disorder, and borderline personality disorder. (These and other disorders will be explained in Chapter 26.) The more disorders a person has, the greater the number of modalities will be required to treat her: day hospitals, inpatient hospital programs, residential treatment centers, more than one individual outpatient psychotherapy session per week, group therapy, and one or more kinds of medications will all be necessary to deal with these other disorders. People who self-injure vary greatly in the degree of their psychological illness.

Self-injury is very treatable. It is more easily treated than the accompanying disorders and their causes.

23

Eating Disorders

The public is, by now, well versed in the topic of eating disorders. Besides the many excellent and widely read books written on this topic since the 1970s, it has been exhaustively covered by articles, documentary news programs, and popular talk shows. Eating disorders continue to fascinate and trouble us.

In this chapter we attempt to narrow the focus of our attention to the relationship between eating disorders and child sexual abuse. Again we remind the reader that many causes can contribute to the development of an eating disorder, the presence of which does not necessarily indicate abuse.

ANOREXIA NERVOSA

As described in Chapter 2, anorexia nervosa is a disorder characterized by an obsession with weight loss; with no goal weight or a continuing lowering of any specified goal weight, as to make goal setting meaningless or insincere. Every thought and behavior involved with weight loss may be employed in the process, from obsessive self-examination and excessive exercise, to the use of laxatives and diuretics ("purging"), to the constant self-accusation that one is too fat when in actuality one may be skeletal. The anorexic has a distorted image of her body: she clings to the idea that she is fat, even though by any objective measure and the opinion of most adults around her she is emaciated. The danger of becoming "even fatter" haunts her.

Anorexia has a poor recovery rate, generally thought to be between 30 and 50 percent. In addition, there is a significant risk of death, even with treatment. According to the *DSM IV* (the fourth edition of the *Diagnostic and Statistical Manual of Mental Disorders* of the American Psychiatric Association), "the long-term mortality from Anorexia Nervosa is over 10%."[7]

Anorexia and childhood sexual abuse The correlation between child sexual abuse and anorexia nervosa is significantly lower than between abuse and self-mutilation. However, approximately half the cutters I have treated or am currently treating were anorexic before turning to self-mutilation. This and other parallels in the development of both anorexia and cutting suggest also looking at anorexia in connection with childhood sexual abuse.

Anorexics, like self-mutilators, may be motivated by different unconscious or conscious emotions. The anorexic may never have developed assertiveness as a child, and as an adolescent may be fearful of expressing anger; anorexia can become the vehicle for that anger. She becomes assertive, even aggressive, with those adults who try to coax her to gain weight. In aspects of her life outside of the defense of her illness, however, she usually has little ability to act assertively. For example, she will defer to others in planning activities, such as which movie to see or where to take a vacation. She is submissive if the issue does not affect her eating, exercise, or weight.

Anorexia nervosa serves many emotional purposes: for those who feel neglected, it can be a way of generating concern from others. It can be a passive-aggressive way to express anger, when the people sufferers are angry with are experienced as dangerous. (*Passive aggression* is a way for a person to deal with her own anger and resentment without having to acknowledge it to herself or express it openly. The passive-aggressive person unconsciously chooses behaviors that provoke others into being angry at her,

while she maintains a demeanor of being compliant and "nice.")
Anorexia can also be a hiding place that distracts the anorexic from
her real fears, fears that relate to potentially harmful people, past
and present.

All of these motives are so deeply unconscious that anorexics
would not be able, nor want, to see such motives as driving their
disorder, which does develop a life of its own and "forgets" its origins. Eating becomes strongly linked with feelings, making food
the target of her fears. By not eating every day, she proves to herself that she can defeat what she fears. If she can do without food,
then she can do without trust and emotional dependency, needs
that showed themselves in her childhood to be too dangerous to try
to meet using the adults around her.

Likewise, the victim of repeated childhood sexual trauma sub-
mitted to the abuse with little or no protest. This is because when
it began, she was powerless and did not believe she had any
recourse to assistance from or protection by others. As she grows
into adolescence, anorexia may provide a sense of protection from
further abuse. In starving away the feminine features of her body,
she hopes to make herself unattractive to those who might assault
her sexually. As malnutrition diminishes her hormone levels, she
also rids herself of her own sex drive.

However, without extensive psychotherapy and often medication, the traumatized survivor may never overcome her fear that
the event will recur. She may never give up obsolete protections,
defense mechanisms, and symptoms resulting from the trauma.
Even if she chooses to become a bodybuilder or a martial arts
expert, her fear of being overpowered by other potential abusers,
even in safe environments, is not likely to go away. More typically,
however, the anorexia will become chronic and she will remain
physically fragile. She has found an area wherein no one can make
her submit—weight gain. Another similarity between anorexics
and survivors of childhood sexual abuse is that both are unable to
pinpoint or reflect on unconscious negative feelings, such as fear
regarding their ability to thrive socially, sexually, maritally, profes-

sionally, or economically in the future. Both groups find it hard to focus on the future or set goals for themselves. For the anorexic, this is probably because of the compelling nature of her obsession with diet and weight. For the abuse survivor, it is due to the belief that future abuse is inevitable (the "forever factor"). Both groups are generally pessimistic about recovering and seem to lack a sense of *agency*, the capacity that enables people to direct their lives and plan a successful future.

Additional characteristics shared by anorexics and survivors of abuse include self-loathing, low self-esteem, and feelings of alienation, which may be masked by a false self (cheery and outgoing). The duration of symptoms is long, sometimes lasting for a lifetime.

Psychotherapy for anorexia   What childhood sexual abuse, self-mutilation, and anorexia all have in common is that sufferers are separated emotionally from others, find it difficult to trust and accept care from others, and have a poor ability to reflect on the deeper reasons for their problems. These patients often resist a therapist's attempts to help them with these aspects of their disorder or problem, either for a long time or for the entire duration of the therapy, which terminates without improvement. This can be intimidating for the therapist; progress is measurable only by weight changes, and the scale is a ticking bomb as far as the medical safety and survival of the patient is concerned.

The time it takes for the patient with an eating disorder to risk talking about real issues is much longer than for the patient whose presenting problems are mood or anxiety disorders. (Both mood and anxiety disorders are described in Chapter 26.) The anorexic also seems less willing to be rid of the disorder or even to modify her symptoms. To "protect" her symptoms she resists talking about them or talking at all in session. This is due to her fear of trust and attachment, as well as feeling that her talk will be inadequate or cause the therapist to think of her as a bad person; it is not hostility. The time frame for developing a therapeutic alliance, or even just plain trust, in the mistrustful patient can take up to a year or longer. Therapist and patient will have to develop a mutual sense of patience with this process.

BULIMIA NERVOSA AND CHILDHOOD SEXUAL ABUSE

Bulimia nervosa is the eating disorder characterized by episodes of bingeing and purging. Once a well-kept secret employed by people to stay thin, it is now widely known and understood by the general public to be a serious problem.

Bulimia is characterized by several distinct features, the first closely related to anorexia—the drive to be thin. Second, during *bingeing*, the bulimic consumes abnormally large quantities of food within a discrete period of time; most binges last two to three hours. Third, in *purging*, the food is eliminated from the body. This can be accomplished in one of several ways: The bulimic may vomit once at the end of the binge or several times throughout the binge. Or she may take an overdose of laxatives, enough to produce diarrhea, so that she can be sure all the ingested food has indeed been purged. Another form of purging is less direct, in that the ingested food is not eliminated, but the bulimic burns up the calories ingested in the binge episode through extreme bouts of physical exercise.

All of these behaviors are potentially addictive because of the chemical changes they create: endorphins result from exercise and bingeing, and laxatives are addictive when taken repeatedly. Psychological dependency on bulimic behavior grows over time, making the addiction both emotional and chemical.

Bulimia, like anorexia, is a dangerous disorder. Repeated vomiting can cause bleeding, even hemorrhaging, in the lining of the gastrointestinal tract. Laxative addiction can weaken or destroy motility of the bowel, so that over time the laxative abuser loses the ability to eliminate naturally.

Bulimia has a negative impact on both self-esteem and emotional coping skills; bulimics use bingeing and purging to handle stress and avoid personal reflection. While eating usually at a faster rate than normal, the bulimic achieves a trancelike state which eliminates awareness of conflict, anxiety, and bad memories. The bulimic who has been sexually abused as a child will use binge/purge episodes to temporarily eradicate memories of abuse. Vomiting has the psychological effect of releasing angry feelings. She may become addicted to this cycle of behavior to prevent the intense feelings which, if they were expressed "normally," she is certain would impair her functioning at school or work.

As with other self-destructive disorders, bulimia should be addressed early in therapy. Since the bulimic often has a normal weight and appearance, therapists tend to overlook the importance of this disorder, regarding it as a symptom of sexual abuse that will resolve itself in time. Because of its addictive quality and emotional significance, bulimia is an important focal point of therapy, whether it emerges before or after a patient discloses her childhood abuse.

Disordered eating is a part of many lives; the disordered behavior serves to disguise or express unresolved emotional conflict. Children who are victims of sexual abuse may find as they grow that some form of eating disorder is the ideal "solution" to their pain.

24

Physical, Sexual, and Social Impairments

I t cannot be repeated too often that victims of childhood sexual abuse face life burdened by their trauma and its aftermath: physical, emotional, and sexual impairments that follow them from childhood to adolescence and on into adulthood. Burdened with guilt that truly belongs to their abuser, they punish themselves with deliberately self-destructive behaviors that affect their femininity, such as anorexia, and "volunteer" to be hurt by other sexual predators. Survivors also mar their bodies by cutting and burning their skin, and then feel shame at the prospect of having a sexual partner see what they have done to themselves. Some survivors fear engaging in sexual activity due to the terrible associations attached to the abuse they suffered when young.

PHYSICAL AND SEXUAL DIFFICULTIES

A number of the women profiled in Part Two can serve as examples of the impairments resulting from childhood sexual abuse. In each of these cases—which we review briefly here—a therapeutic alliance and consistent treatment were needed before the survivor could overcome her damaging legacy.

Doreen   In Doreen's case, a cruel brother and indifferent family led to a combination of physical and sexual impairments. As a young adult she was still living at home, and though her older brother was no longer abusing her sexually, he was hurting her physically. Now, as when she was a young child being sexually abused by him, her parents were indifferent to her complaints about his behavior, favoring her older brother in disputes and providing her with little emotional support.

Because of the sexual abuse, she had learned to fuse pain with sexual arousal. She developed relationships with sadistic men, in which she could only be aroused by experiencing various forms pain, which she directed her partner to give her during sex. Moreover, her masochistic desire for painful stimulation was escalating toward levels that were dangerous for her health and life. In addition to her sexual dysfunction with men, she developed the physical compulsion to scratch herself (on her arms, chest, and face), and this, too, evolved into a form of private sexual gratification for her.

June   Earlier, in discussing June (Chapter 3) we saw her childhood legacy limited her to behavior in relationships that made her very unhappy and lowered her self-esteem. June's brother's behavior was a mixture of support, abuse, and seduction. June had absentee parents who did not notice the abuse. But she was not suffering from the severe trauma that Doreen experienced when she came to therapy, and so was able to strive for success in the business world and to develop skills that brought her high-paying jobs. June could also communicate that she required respect from men in professional (though not in personal) relationships. June's romantic life was dismal and as a teen she had developed anorexia. As an adult she suffered socially and was taken advantage of and treated badly in romantic relationships. Because of the childhood abuse she did not feel entitled to anything better.

Olivia   Like Doreen, Olivia (Chapter 12) had a different legacy. She had developed a mechanism referred to as *conversion hysteria*, in which the brain alters the way the body functions, affecting its ability to send and receive messages from parts of her body. In her case she became vaginally anesthetized. Her brain disallowed sexual arousal since arousal originated from assault, which she interpreted as assault even as a child when it was happening.

Gina   Due to the massive nature of sexual assaults by her father and brothers, Gina developed an extremely aggressive posture toward men in order to manage her fear of them. She became a lesbian most likely because that seemed the only safe haven from the cruelty she had endured. She also protected herself and kept her sexuality alive by taking on the male role in relationships. By choosing the same object (female) her father and her brothers had done, she was identifying with the power of the males who had attacked her, albeit without the assaultive behavior. The primary goal of her treatment would not be to make her become a heterosexual woman, but to free her of the defensive fear, aggressive behavior, and hatred of men that tormented her and sabotaged her ability to find her place in work and her social life.

Ava   Ava's father was sexually sadistic with her when she was young; he used his belt buckle and other objects to penetrate and hurt her. She developed a fear of vaginal contamination from these objects. When she reached puberty and started menstruating, the menses, in her view, symbolized proof of the contamination of her vagina. Before puberty she would wash the area until it was irritated. Menstruation brought fear of toxic shock syndrome (a rare but potentially fatal illness that has been associated with tampon use) and the possibilities of vaguely defined infections, though she was not sexually active. She began to put rubbing alcohol into her vagina. She reasoned that this would make her bacterially sterile and protect her from contamination.

In therapy we discussed the symbolic meaning of washing away the memories of her abuse with the alcohol. I sent her to a gyne-cologist, who explained that using alcohol internally on vaginal tis-sue disrupted and damaged the internal environment of the mucous membrane. She was told that this kind of cleansing would make her vulnerable to infection and that the body produced its own "cleaning fluids," like lactic acid. But Ava only increased her application of the alcohol. The result was dryness and discomfort during and after sex, making sex difficult to enjoy for physical rea-sons alone. It seemed that she was reenacting the pain and survival of her father assaults. She also applied the alcohol after sex to wash the man's fluids out of her body, causing still more pain.

The pain became her emotional safety. Like Doreen, Ava had fused sex with pain. However, in Ava's case the physical discomfort created by the alcohol cleansing eventually drove away her sexual partners; subsequently she substituted cocaine for sex. Ava had inadvertently taken her father's place as her own abuser. She needed to learn to reframe the meaning of sex. This would take a long time since its meaning had been perverted by her father's behavior early in her childhood. She also had to become educated about the female body and familiar with her own body in order to dispel myths she held and to become willing to stop using the harmful physical remedies she had adopted to treat her psychological pain.

Physical impairments to sexual function Even if the original abuse has not physically injured the child's body enough to create sexual impairment in adulthood, the psychological damage done by the abuse may lead her, as an adolescent or adult, to choose sexual activities that damage her body. Doreen, reviewed earlier in the chapter, is one example. Another is Annie (Chapter 5). Annie suf-fered from physical discomfort during any sort of penetration due to the damage done during a period when she had engaged in exhi-bitionistic, masochistic sex, often with multiple partners at the same time. She then entered into a relationship with Gina. When the two women met, Annie was recovering from surgery to repair internal tissues injured during her reckless, multipartner days.

Physical impairments to sexual functioning can also stem from anxiety associated with sexual contacts. Again, Annie and Gina provide an example: each woman had a prior history involving physically violent sex. Gina had had been raped as a child by several members of her family at one time. In Annie's case, masochistic sex with men was "voluntary," but she was always drunk during these encounters. Alcoholism, usually connected to her sexual exploits, emerged early in therapy as one of Annie's problems. She could not recall ever having had sex—before being with Gina—unless she was inebriated. When the two women became involved, they both got sober. Now they were anxious about sex and shy with each other in bed. In general, anxiety about sex inhibits both arousal and orgasm, making intimacy uncomfortable. In addition, despite the lack of violence they had difficulty receiving pleasure: each refused to be the receiver of sexual touching by the other.

SOCIAL HANDICAPS

As the stories in this book attest, the negative impacts of childhood sexual abuse proliferate far beyond the physical and sexual damage. Personality limitations—including distancing others, being overly aggressive, isolating oneself socially, and showing inappropriate extroversion (indiscreet overexposure of the body)—can cause victims to lose relationships with friends and lovers.

Social handicaps are most pronounced during the teenage years, when other girls begin talking about boys and the survivor of childhood sexual abuse shies away from taking an active part in the conversation. She seldom dates and does not let a physical relationship with a boy develop, because she equates sexual behavior with victimization. Deirdre (in Chapter 4) is an example of this social handicap: she became a wallflower. When the survivor's friends compare notes, she does not participate. Instead she drops away from her friendship group since she does not share their excitement over their new adventures. She begins to feel different and inferior from the group and her self-esteem drops—she develops self-loathing and feels alienated. She may channel these feelings into cutting or other self-contained methods of emotional relief, such as anorexia and/or bulimia.

If the abuse survivor does not become socially withdrawn, she may simply act as "one of the guys," abandoning her feminine identity in a coed situation. She talks about sports or gives platonic advice to boys about succeeding with girls. Over time, the friendships of abused girls who adopt this social demeanor become increasingly shallow. She also has her secret that she cannot share with her friends. This understandably makes her feel different and may drive her into depression or further into self-harming behavior. Michelle, for example, who had been fondled by her fifth grade teacher, told no one; she coped as a teenager by becoming pals with the boys on the baseball team and was accepted as their sidekick. Sadly, the survivor's friends allow her to drift away; they do not see her inner unhappiness and disorder.

As this pattern solidifies she may develop more difficulty with life decisions, such as choosing a college (if she's college-bound) or thinking about work and her future in general. As a patient once said to me when asked about thoughts on her future, "I can't think beyond today. I have less and less sense of who I am and where I belong. Probably I just belong alone. Sure, I'll have friends and get along with people, but my sense of loneliness and the absence of closeness to anyone—it grows and bothers me increasingly. Sometimes I have suicidal thoughts, though I guess I won't act on them."

Social handicaps deriving from childhood sexual abuse center for the most part on isolation and feelings of alienation. These and other traits limit the social success the abuse survivor could have had if she had not been victimized as a child.

In this chapter, we reviewed a variety of physical, sexual, and social impairments resulting from childhood sexual abuse. We also described the underlying emotional damage, including depression and low self-esteem, which can both cause and result from sexual dysfunction.

Throughout Part Three, the focus has been on understanding the legacy of abuse in its various manifestations. With the knowledge gained from these chapters, as well as from Parts One and Two, we turn now to consider recovery: what kinds of treatment or treatments are helpful, and how does a good therapeutic relationship work to repair the damage and improve the survivor's relationships with herself and others?

PART FOUR

■

RECOVERING
STOLEN
TOMORROWS

25

Developing Readiness
for Treatment

C hange is the goal for most therapy, and change is difficult. We are all more comfortable with the familiar, even when society deems it unhealthy or self-destructive. Survivors of childhood abuse are especially challenged in the therapeutic setting because of their intense issues around trust and disclosure. With many patients the first stage of therapy has to center on developing *readiness*, the willingness to open up and to want change.

ADDRESSING SYMPTOMATIC BEHAVIORAL DISORDERS

Most patients who have survived childhood sexual abuse come to psychotherapy presenting problems like those described in earlier chapters—post-traumatic stress disorder, eating disorders, and anxiety disorders. (An *anxiety disorder* is characterized by excessive, hard-to-control worry, which affects sleep, concentration, mood, and energy levels. Unlike a phobia, which has a specific target, the anxiety can be generalized and interferes with socializing and functioning at school or work.) They have difficulty wanting to relinquish the behaviors and symptoms they associate with emotional safety, though they feel an obligation to try. For example, Maureen (whom we met in Chapter 15) was attached to her bulimia because she relied on it to soothe her distress. It took courage for her to relinquish what therapists view as a disorder but what felt to her like an ally, and was a mainstay of her emotional life.

Compounding this resistance to giving up self-destructive behaviors is the combination of personality traits many abuse survivors bring to therapy: nurturing, caretaking, and people pleasing. Survivors are often reluctant to be receivers of care, support, reassurance, and assistance. They are polite, self-effacing, and apologetic with little ability to be confronting or provocative in a straightforward manner. Beneath their pleasant, agreeable, helpful demeanor, however, lie fear, suspicion, anger, and low self-esteem. These patients are not complainers. A therapist who is looking for the patient who will complain and vent on the first session will be disappointed. During the early stages of treatment, "waiting the patient out with silence" will cause her to leave treatment fast. So will asking her directly why she is caught up in the behavior that led her to seek treatment; she will perceive the therapist as ignorant and weak, much as a medical patient might view a physician who asks a patient why she has a fever.

Questions that begin "What . . . ?" or "How long . . . ?" will be acceptable to the patient, as long as they are accompanied by the therapist explaining her disorder and its symptoms to her. In addition, the therapist must demonstrate knowledge of the kinds of feelings, beliefs, and personality traits she is likely to have. These statements will give the therapist credibility in the patient's eyes as someone capable of understanding her. No therapist is a mind reader, but when a patient discloses a symptomatic behavior pattern, the therapist should comment with generalizations based on statements shared by other patients with her pattern.

For example, we know many of the thoughts, feelings, and rituals of anorexics. These are some common statements made in early sessions:

"If I don't have anorexia, I won't have anything."

"If I start eating, I'll never be able to stop and I'll wind up obese."

"I don't care what the scale says—I know I've gained weight."

"When people tell me I look good, I get angry because I know it means that I'm not thin enough."

"I think that when people say I look good they mean I'm fat."

Common statements made by self-mutilators are:

"Cutting is the only thing that can stop the anxiety."

"If I don't cut myself, I won't stop thinking about it until I do."

"I have to see the blood—then I'm okay."

"I thought I'd stopped hurting myself but—it's back."

Expressions of fear and admissions of compulsive behaviors will come later, as treatment progresses.

Viewed dispassionately, these early statements are part of her unconscious goal to distance and even provoke the therapist. If the therapist becomes frustrated with the patient (and many therapists do), she will sense this and then will feel "safe" from having to develop trust, dependency, or closeness.

The same elements exist in the adolescent or adult woman who has not resolved her issues about childhood abuse. She, too, has painted people around her with the broad brush of danger. Her early statements may be subtler than those of the anorexic or self-cutter—if she is not also an anorexic (or former anorexic). Regardless, her perception of safety lies in the separation between herself and others. She does not want to be transparent to them.

BREAKING THROUGH THE SURVIVOR'S
PROTECTIVE SHELL

By the time a patient with a history of childhood sexual abuse
enters therapy, she may have told her story to others, including
other therapists. When she tells these stories, she generally hides
any signs of her true feelings about the abuse from her listener and
from herself. She separates herself from her reactions and feelings
connected to the events that she is describing. She does this to
avoid the possibility of flashbacks, which force her to relive the fear
and pain of the original events. Each time she enters a therapist's
office for the first time, she risks this vulnerability: she does not
want the therapist to break through the defenses that protect her
from having a flashback. Psychotherapy requires trust and vulnerability, and this new patient has no positive associations with these
qualities. In fact, she dreads them; in her experience they lead to
assault. The therapist's task is akin to convincing an acrophobic that
it would be fun to walk a tightrope without a net.

Addressing a patient with trauma in her background   Years
ago it was common practice for psychiatrists to ask direct questions
about trauma—such as "Have you ever been sexually abused?"—in
the first session. The problem with asking the new patient this sort
of question early on is that she will answer in a detached or dissociated state, the same detachment she used when coping with her
abuser. Her tone may be matter-of-fact, but she is definitely not
relating to her questioner in the present. That the psychiatrist got
the information prematurely just makes it more difficult to volun-
tarily revisit that information when it would be therapeutic to do so.
In a trusting relationship, getting to statements of the abuse is a
slow and painful process. Her account of sexual abuse must be volunteered at first, and in future sessions elicited sensitively, with
constant attention paid to what the patient will tolerate emotionally. The experienced and intuitive therapist observes behavioral
cues ranging from timidity or lack of femininity to extreme flirta-

tiousness, even seductiveness. When the patient presents these cues early in therapy she is signaling that abuse has occurred and is probably ready to discuss it.

Thus, with a patient who has trauma in her background, the first task of the therapist is to move slowly toward the goal of creating a relationship in which she sees the therapist as her nurturer. Generally, the therapist has to approach her as if invited to do so. To do this, the therapist has to see past her defense of distancing and believe that she wants to be reached, even though it will be emotionally uncomfortable for her. This places special demands on the therapist. Among them is not to be "wounded" by the patient, moreover, to risk liking this resistant and rejecting person. She is just not ready yet. The process takes time. A year of sessions is not an especially long time for her to decide it is safe for her to begin using the therapist as a trusted and guiding person.

Maureen's case illustrates explicitly how all of the above can happen. Maureen certainly did not need to begin therapy by reviewing her early traumatic events and would have become angry had I mistakenly asked her to do so. What she needed, more than historical analysis or interpretation, were "here and now tools" she could accept from someone she trusted and to whom she felt attached. Maureen's job in therapy, which is ongoing, was and is to use the therapist to help her develop mental skills to "regulate" her flashbacks, so she can gradually put them in perspective as "bad memories." This will also help give her more faith in her ability to deal with fear or worry in healthy ways, to give up seeking relief through old defenses, such as bulimic episodes of bingeing and vomiting.

Taking care to develop trust Survivors of childhood sexual abuse are rightfully the least trusting people a therapist will encounter. Even if this patient seems pleasant and cooperative, it does not mean real trust and attachment in a therapeutic alliance is going to be easy to develop. It is important to be aware of the profundity of this patient's inexperience with trust, fear of trust, contempt of trust, even disbelief in its existence—all of which makes a helping relationship very difficult. Many a well-meaning therapist has lost a patient after assuming a trust that did not exist. Just as often, a patient may have unexpressed disillusionment with her therapist; regarding him or her as trying hard but not succeeding in understanding her core issues.

Thus before a therapist can use any degree of authority to encourage behavioral change in the patient and to assist her in altering the way she relates to herself emotionally, the therapist must have done a lot of "nurturing homework" to earn that level of trust. This homework consists of listening empathically, validating the patient's feelings, and spelling out why and how self-destructive behaviors develop as a response to abuse. For a patient to tolerate a therapist's authoritative behavior, no matter how subtle, requires an extraordinary level of trust on her part. When that has occurred, wonderful changes will develop.

If an authoritative stance is employed too early in the process, the patient's reaction is immediate transference: "Hey, you're not my parent!" Moreover, a parent may have molested her. Nothing therapeutic will happen.

In addition to not being directly authoritative (like a parent) too soon, the therapist must take care not to behave in a way that the patient could interpret as being seductive, like a potential abuser (with no bad intent but too warm and "touch-feely"), or like someone who would take advantage of the patient's vulnerability by acting on his or her own mental sexual agenda regarding the patient. The patient will be hypersensitive to this, making her inaccessible to treatment with this therapist. (For reasons mentioned earlier, the patient may behave provocatively and seductively either as a testing device or simply because this is her characteristic social posture when meeting new people.)

When the therapist does his or her "nurturing homework," the therapist's authoritative behavior can be incorporated by the patient who will then feel protected, not bullied.

In the beginning of a therapeutic relationship the therapist needs to understand and state a number of things to the patient:

One is acknowledge that this is not a comfortable undertaking for her. Another is to warn her that even with the best match of personalities, a strong motivation on her part to heal, and a skillful therapist, treatment is likely to be long and uneven. Each person will need to be patient and ask that same patience from the other. Do not state that treatment for those who were sexually abused as children is impossible, just that it is complicated and difficult. Emphasize (as illustrated in this book) that it can have successful outcomes.

THE SIGNIFICANCE OF GENDER

When the therapist is of a different gender than the perpetrator, this lessens the likelihood that the patient will transfer suspicion of an assault to the therapist. On the other hand, many girls who were molested by their fathers become angry with their mothers first. Whether expressed verbally or not, these patients think, "I know he's crazy but she should have been aware enough to protect me from him."

For example, for Cassie (Chapter 11), it was the emergence of her mother's face on her paintings that brought back memories of her father assaulting her. Recall what Cassie stated: "[My mother] even allowed him to move his bed away from hers, right near the doorway so he could easily slip out in the middle of the night to rape me." Cassie saw women as competitors and as being nonprotective of her. She reacted negatively to the female therapist she saw before coming to see me. When I asked Cassie why she left her first therapist, Cassie's response was vague. Eventually she stated that she just didn't trust women.

A different female patient might have never taken a chance on a male therapist. The point is not to generalize that one gender of therapist is preferable for treating childhood sexual abuse, but to point out that if gender is an issue, it should be explored early in therapy.

26

Setting Therapeutic Goals

In the emotionally fraught context of childhood sexual abuse and its resulting effects on the psyche, therapy must set goals in order to provide structure, thereby preventing the therapeutic relationship from becoming derailed. Goals relating to psychological, physical, or sexual, and social development have to be discussed with the patient, and agreed on early in treatment. In the following pages we take a look at how therapy addresses the symptoms of various disorders and other impairments. We begin with the most serious in terms of danger to the patient, moving on to conditions that are decreasingly life-threatening.

RELIEF FROM PSYCHOSIS

The first goal to establish is getting the patient relief from the symptoms of any of several mental disorders that may be present. The most serious of these disorders is *psychosis*, which consists of mental activity resulting in thoughts and feelings that are inconsistent with reality or grossly inappropriate to a given situation. Psychotic behavior and speech may seem extremely "unreasonable."

Another term currently in use, in addition to "psychotic phenomena," is *dissociative disorders*, examples of which have been mentioned previously. They include *dissociative identity disorder* (formerly *multiple personality disorder*) and *dissociative amnesia disorder*. More extensive descriptions of these can be found in the *DSM IV*.

Psychotic episodes are treated by a combination of psychotherapy and antipsychotic medication prescribed by a psychiatrist.

In addition to patients who may need relief for an ongoing psychosis, some patients exhibit little or no psychotic behavior in sessions until discussions of the original sexual abuse come up. At this point, they may become lost in "chaos," becoming truly incomprehensible in their verbal and nonverbal responses. The therapist's task at that point is to calm the patient down. When therapist and patient have known each other long enough for the "healthy" part of the patient to trust the therapist, she will be accessible to comments and suggestions by the therapist that will bring her out of the psychotic state. The therapist's calming talk will induce her out of the mental chaos of a psychotic episode.

If a trusting relationship between therapist and patient has not had time to develop, or if the therapist lacks skill in dealing with this kind of psychotic episode, the therapist may need to call in medical staff or EMT personnel to sedate the patient. Sedation is the least desirable alternative to coping with the episode, unless she is a clear danger to herself or others, because it represents a lost opportunity to encourage the patient to be less afraid of her mind by using the therapist's confidence in her; forced sedation may also weaken the therapeutic relationship. Nevertheless, there are times when therapists have to call for physical and chemical support. Julie's story (Chapter 17) is an example of such a case.

RELIEF FROM MOOD DISORDERS

The second goal is the alleviation of *mood disorders*. These include depression, *dysthymia* (a combination of depression and anxiety), and *bipolar disorder* (formerly referred to as manic depressive disorder, or simply *manic depression*, and characterized by severe mood swings).

Relief from mood disorders is vital to the treatment for child-hood sexual abuse since they can all contribute to self-harming behavior (including self-mutilation). Mood disorders also cause lowered self-esteem and self-loathing, which in turn leave the patient vulnerable to predatory and exploitative persons. Left untreated, a person who has been victimized in the past could be taken advantage of in both sexual and nonsexual ways.

These disorders respond well to medication when used in con-junction with psychotherapy. The decision to use medication is sen-sitive; many patients prefer not to use psychotropic medicine, or they need time to consider it without being pressured. (*Psychotropic medicine*, also called *psychiatric medication*, is drugs that have an altering effect on the mind, such as antidepressants or tranquilizers.) The therapist needs to be attuned to the patient's readiness for medication, and to individually assess the risks and benefits of taking or not taking medication for each patient.

Two of the case studies given in Part Two offer examples of treat-ing mood disorders in survivors of childhood sexual abuse: Marjorie for depression, and Audrey for bipolar disorder. Let's con-sider their cases again.

Marjorie (Chapter 7) was so defeated by the abuse she had expe-rienced at the hands of her Uncle Bill that she lapsed into passivity when boys she dated groped her, assumed her baby daughter would grow up to prefer her husband over her as the more valuable parent, and in general suffered from depression and pessimism about herself. The experience of childhood sexual abuse created a view of her place in the world, a world where she would always be a victim, losing out in life in terms of achievement and respect. Treating her depression involved role playing and practicing con-versations so she could develop assertiveness and overcome her fear of others being angry or dissatisfied with her.

During our role playing, I would typically play Marjorie and she would play the person she felt unable to confront or to request something from. We worked on body posture, body language, and use of her voice. She was given assignments to try out new ways of behaving with others when opportunities to do so arose in between sessions. She was to "act as if" she really felt the underlying confidence appropriate to these new behaviors, even though at first they felt foreign to her. We would discuss these incidents afterwards. She discovered that each time she was able to try out a new behavior and it worked successfully, she became a little more confident. As other people responded positively to her fake assertiveness, it became real, and thus a new facet of her personality developed.

In addition to receiving psychotherapy, Marjorie was prescribed an antidepressant to combat the chemical alteration the abuse had effected in her brain. The combination of medicine and psychotherapy was far more effective than psychotherapy would have been alone. At the time, we did not know whether the medication would be temporary or permanent. She was given the option of stopping her medication after a few months, a year, or longer—whenever it became clear it could safely be eliminated.

The focus of therapy continued to be the enhancement of Marjorie's self-esteem and confidence. She developed a sense of empowerment as a parent and felt like an equal partner in her marriage. Today Marjorie and her husband have three healthy children and she is a part-time manager of a computer store. As of this writing, she is still taking a mild antidepressant drug, which she will continue until she is no longer impaired by self-doubt.

In the case of Audrey (Chapter 13), her characteristic behavior in therapy consisted of alternating between intense bouts of crying and loud, rapid talk interlaced with angry cursing. She felt mistreated by family members and boyfriends, and alienated from the world of work, which she could not cope with. When Audrey lost her seven-year position as the assistant to a wealthy philanthropist, she did not have the financial resources to afford a place to live on her own, and she felt crushed by having to return to the comparative poverty and low status of living in her mother's apartment. The years of living in her philanthropist-benefactor's opulent triplex apartment had given her notions of grandeur and made it extremely difficult for her to get a sense of who she was and where she belonged. Negative feelings about work would alternate with high hopes that she could become a famous actor. She would go to a few acting classes but then start skipping them, sinking into the negative feelings that brought a halt to her progress. She would then slide back to drug-addicted boyfriends with whom she would get high.

The rapid changes in her mood, characteristic of bipolar disorder, made it impossible for Audrey to follow through on any plan she made for her life. She was given medication to treat bipolar disorder, as well as an antidepressant. Leveling her extreme highs and lows assisted the psychotherapy by helping her to focus on reality. Audrey's emotional patterns are still quite extreme and will probably require medication for a long time, and possibly permanently.

RELIEF FROM ANXIETY DISORDERS

The third category of disorders, highly represented in childhood sexual abuse, is *anxiety disorders*. These include generalized anxiety disorder and obsessive-compulsive disorder. Each of these can serve as a refuge from memories and flashbacks, but they tend to eventually block out many nontraumatic recollections as well. People with these disorders may experience their anxiety directly as *anxiety attacks* (severe, intensely uncomfortable episodes of fear). Or they may experience it indirectly, though unconsciously, by causing some body part to malfunction (producing, for example, hysterical blindness or digestive distress).

Experiencing *undefined anxiety* (or free-floating anxiety, in which the person feels nervous but does not know why) is usually the most emotionally painful state for a child who has been sexually abused to experience because she lacks a strategy to make it go away. This anxiety can be extremely intense, as the child struggles with her fear and helplessness. The lack of protection from the abuse generates in the child a need for a self-contained "system" of emotional safety—in others words, a hiding place. In adolescence undefined anxiety often emerges in the form of one or more addictive or compulsive behavior disorders, such as anorexia or self-mutilation. Thus our list of goals must also include recovery from any of these that may be present: self-mutilation (cutting and/or burning), eating disorders (anorexia nervosa, bulimia nervosa, and compulsive overeating), obsessive-compulsive disorder (OCD), and drug and/or alcohol abuse. Because of their potentially severe, life-threatening nature, the first two of these three groups were covered in depth earlier in the book (Chapters 22 and 23). OCD, which does not occur frequently in conjunction with childhood sexual abuse, was briefly discussed in Chapter 2.

As discussed in Chapter 2, most anorexics suffer from anxieties and develop ritualistic behaviors to combat them that resemble obsessive-compulsive disorders. However, these behaviors are not usually indicative of true OCD unless they are not related to food, weight, body shape, or body size. In anorexia, the primary disorder is a generalized anxiety disorder, which initially centers on dieting, but expands to include other weight-loss behaviors, such as the use of laxatives and excessive exercise, which overlap with bulimia as well.

For our purposes, we are looking at anorexia as an emotional hiding place where the victim can forget her childhood sexual abuse and its resultant severe insecurity; there is no one available for protection. Anorexia also serves to channel the anxiety stemming from the childhood sexual abuse to a manageable, though self-destructive, set of symptoms that often evolve into an intractable disorder. It is yet another example of how childhood sexual abuse spawns clusters of emotional disorders that must be treated along with the original trauma.

In therapy, the discussion must eventually transition from anorexia, bulimia, cutting, or other anxiety-disorder symptoms to the abuse, which was the original trauma. Awareness of the details of abuse will vary in content and level of feeling. Some patients can tell stories about the abuse, while others describe fragmented flashbacks that were intense and might throw them into dissociated states during a therapy session. A minority of patients become ver-bally withdrawn, or else act out with shouting, intense crying, and verbal threats. Occasionally a patient has a psychotic episode. If this happens, it is appropriate for the therapist to respond as described earlier in the chapter (in the section "Relief from Psychosis").

RELIEF FROM PHYSICAL AND/OR SEXUAL IMPAIRMENTS

Goals of treatment must also include relief from any physical symp-toms that can accompany trauma. These include bodily pain, invol-untary muscular contractions, sensations of burning, pain, immobility, problems involving the autonomic (involuntary) nerv-ous system, digestive problems, tachycardia (episodes of rapid heartbeat), and others. Many of these symptoms combine with damage done to the survivor's sexuality, including always experienc-ing arousal fused with pain and choosing dangerous physical behav-iors during the sex act.

Another important therapeutic goal is to relieve any sexual hand-icaps or dysfunctions the patient may have. Pain due to physical malfunctioning, or even just the inability to perform sexually, can generate a fear of sexual activity, which in turn threatens the healthy sexual relationship the victim is trying to establish in her adult life.

See Chapter 24 for more discussion of physical and sexual impairments.

RELIEF FROM SOCIAL CONSEQUENCES

Survivors of childhood abuse can be extremely shy and awkward in social situations, hampered by low self-esteem and may feel secretly stigmatized by their history. In other cases, the opposite behaviors occur, resulting in sexual aggressiveness and compulsive seduction. Learning to make different, healthier choices in relationships—such as avoiding harmful, assaultive, and exploitative men and women—is a critically important task in therapy. This is best accomplished through interpretation (in which the therapist helps the patient understand the feelings, motivations, and significance surrounding her choices) and by doing exercises, such as role playing and developing scripts, among others.

The survivor is entitled to be free of her self-damaging behaviors, negative thoughts and ideas, and mood disorders, which, when untreated, will sabotage and limit her choices, success, and happiness.

27

Balancing Bonding
with Boundaries

Therapy is a delicate relationship because it must weather a wide range of feelings and often volatile reactions. The connection between patient and therapist has to remain constant throughout the stormy process of moving from discovery to understanding, from pain to healing. To maintain this consistent connection requires genuine caring on the one hand, while maintaining appropriate boundaries on the other.

TRANSFERENCE, COUNTERTRANSFERENCE, AND CARING

Relationships that help an individual to change are personal, whether they take place in a professional setting, such as psychotherapy, or in friendships, romances, and marriages. This has always been a difficult issue to address in psychotherapy. When is "personal" or "caring" helpful, and when does it become a liability? Psychotherapists protect themselves by labeling patients' feelings toward them "transference" and their own feelings toward patients as "countertransference." These concepts help keep the therapeutic process balanced and reasonable, even when dealing with the highly charged and challenging issue of sexual abuse and its aftermath. They also protect the patient and therapist from chaos by establishing emotional and behavioral boundaries on both their parts.

Transference consists of the feelings a patient may develop toward the therapist which come (are "transferred") from her past history dealing with other people who may resemble the therapist in his or her position of authority. The patient usually considers the therapist an authority figure, as she would a parent, teacher, doctor, clergyman, or similar person. She develops attitudes, positive or negative, as if she were dealing with that other person. It is up to the therapist to identify transference when it occurs, and to explain it to the patient; otherwise the therapist may inadvertently reenact one of the patient's past relationships. If this is not discussed with her, it will leave her conflict unimproved or even worsened.

Countertransference represents those feelings and ideas from the therapist's own past that emerge in sessions when a patient's behavior or personality resembles someone significant to the therapist. If the therapist does not recognize that he or she is "misplacing" such feelings onto the patient, the therapist is likely to misunderstand and probably mistreat the patient in word, attitude, or behavior.

Being mindful of the patient's transference and careful to monitor countertransference provide boundaries and discretion in the delicate relationship of therapy. Therapy with inadequate boundaries can cause one of several kinds of inappropriate situations to develop: One is *rescuers syndrome*, in which the therapist feels personally responsible for saving the patient from the world or from herself. Or the therapy could evolve into an overly casual relationship, like a friendship, or worst of all, a romance. Any of these developments will cause therapy to suffer and most likely be ineffective in helping the patient achieve recovery. On the other hand, the therapist must also genuinely care about the patient in order for therapy to be "real" enough to help. Too much detachment will produce a cold, intellectualized therapy, which, like too much closeness, is useless to the patient. Therapists in general, but especially those treating disorders resulting from sexual abuse, must be mindful of the need both to be caring and to maintain boundaries. This is a complicated dilemma for psychotherapists.

A CLOSER LOOK AT TRANSFERENCE

When therapy starts, transference begins to develop: the patient starts transferring her feelings and needs from past experiences with authoritative figures—chiefly her parents, but also including teachers, doctors, ministers, older siblings, and other older relatives such as aunts, uncles, and grandparents—onto the therapist. These feelings include affection and a need for attachment and dependency, but also, fear, shame, and anger. The patient unconsciously transfers these emotions onto the therapist because she perceives him or her to be an authority figure. Because of this transference the patient has expectations of this new relationship; these expectations vary, molded by a patient's individual childhood experiences. When the patient first meets the therapist, her conscious feelings toward him or her may be neutral, but unconsciously she is anticipating a re-creation of these past experiences. The patients we are discussing here anticipate abuse. The transference for the first-time patient will be most intense.

It is important to distinguish between the patient who has never disclosed childhood sexual abuse to anyone and the patient who previously disclosed her abuse to one or more persons—therapists or people she is close to. This is because the needs of patients in these two groups differ in the early sessions. The previously undisclosed patient comes to therapy for some reason other than childhood sexual abuse. The most common is self-mutilation. She uses the initial sessions, before she has disclosed the abuse, as a way to evaluate the therapist in terms of trustworthiness. This may be partly a conscious process and partly an unconscious exploration. Having never disclosed these experiences, she is tense during these sessions, likely to come late or skip appointments without knowing why. If she has repressed her memories of her abuse, she may become aware of her abuse when enough trust has been achieved during the course of therapy. If she was already aware of the abuse before coming to therapy, she may be unsure whether she wants to disclose it or not. She may be embarrassed about it or concerned that the therapist will judge her negatively; she fears that she will be seen as a bad person. If the therapist is nonjudgmental about symptoms such as cutting or starving, the required trust will develop.

The patient who has discussed her abuse with previous therapists or other people evaluates her new therapist more consciously in order to decide whether he or she can become trustworthy.

In either case, transference will occur as the therapy proceeds. In some cases the transference develops gradually along the path created by the expectations the patient had of her abusers. Often this involves duplicating the feelings she had toward her abuser and the way she coped with him—even if the therapist behaves nothing like that person. This type of transference emerged strongly in the case of Melissa.

Melissa: A case of strong transference   I recall her, an incest survivor, sitting on the couch at perhaps her second session, making seductive poses. When I ignored her body language, she said, "If you came over and sat next to me on this couch, I don't think I could stop you from doing anything to me."

"Are you referring to sexual behavior?"

"Um hmm," she nodded.

"That would be abusive toward you," I responded. "And there's no abuse permitted in this relationship."

She seemed uncomfortable. "What would you do if I walked over to you and grabbed your pecker?"

Surprised at her aggressive threat, I responded with "I would know that you had lost control of yourself and that you hoped your aggressiveness would bring a response from me that would put you in a more familiar situation—such as me behaving sexually toward you or getting angry. But that wouldn't happen. I would tell you to calm down and sit down."

She seemed lost and embarrassed. "Don't you think I'm pretty?"

"That has nothing to do with it. This is a therapy session, not an encounter that would reinforce what has happened to you repeatedly in the past."

"But you would like to?" She was trying to negotiate.

"If I say no, does that make you feel lost and powerless?"

She smiled, ambivalent about whether to continue with her attempt to seduce me or admit what was behind her behavior. Finally she sighed and coolly said, "Yeah, I guess so."

Melissa was angry with me for disempowering her. She was not ready to give up the seductive identity she had learned as a child at the hands of her father. She had nothing to replace it with. She also feared that if I did not desire her, I would have no other reason to be interested in her. I told her that she had much strength and that made her an interesting person.

"I don't know what you mean by 'much strength,' but I know it's not as important as being wanted, desired."

"Your most important strength will always be your sexual prowess?"

She nodded vigorously.

"What if I'm not interested in you sexually but I find you an interesting personality?"

"Then you're a fool," she giggled.

"Is that because *you* don't think you're interesting?"

She stopped smiling. "I know what I'm good for . . . and what I'm not."

"Maybe you don't know enough about yourself, only what you've been taught by your father and have gotten other men to verify."

"Well, let me tell you, there's been *a lot* of verifyin'." She looked at once triumphant and degraded.

"Do you think you can find the strength to continue to come here without that 'verifyin'?"

She seemed to like the challenge and offered me a defiant nod.

Due to her transference, Melissa had expected sexual abuse to be part of her therapy relationship. When that didn't occur, she was disoriented and experienced emotions ranging from anger to worthlessness. In subsequent sessions she realized that her seductive and promiscuous behavior was a compulsion; she did not get any enjoyment from it but felt compelled to act that way. It was a major insight for her to see her behavior as a symptom of her childhood abuse and not as "the most valuable part of her." She abandoned nearly all her seductive behavior in the office; her initial transference had changed from expecting sexual abuse to expecting therapeutic help.

Melissa's life was changing outside the office as well. She channeled more of her energy into her business and paid more attention to her daughter. Her marriage had suffered from frequent affairs prompted by her sexual compulsion. As she began to understand the emotional origin of her seductiveness, Melissa began to work out her relationship with her husband.

That early session did not change or eliminate what had been more than twenty years of reaction and adjustment to her abuse, but it clearly identified Melissa's problems. Together we agreed that whenever she behaved that way in session I would identify it and we would interpret why she had reverted to this behavior. The trigger for her seductiveness might be the subject we were talking about, or it could be my expression of interest as she spoke, which she interpreted as being flirtatious or indicating desire. The continuous conscious attention we paid to her seductive or flirtatious moments slowly whittled them down.

Our interpretations eventually became a cause for light humor between us. She made fun of her seductive moments, and the drama and need for them diminished. Following is an example of a humorous exchange, but notice that the lightness also allowed stronger feelings to emerge.

"Are you causing your skirt to ride up?"

"You're no fun at all. Seeing a little thigh might liven you up."

"What would it do for you?"

"Screw me up and set me back I guess. Hey, does this mean I should wear ankle-length skirts and join a nunnery? Shouldn't I ever be sexy?"

"Yes, if you know what you're doing, and why, and with whom."

"Oh, now you're going to make me faithful to my husband," she paused. "Okay, I have been faithful to my husband, and yes, sex has been fun for a change. I feel like those alcoholics that count their days of sobriety. But I admit it's getting easier. I think I'm less fearful about my marriage breaking up or my daughter finding out about the dark side of me. I still wish I could get even with my father for what he did to me, but if I took him to court the whole town would find out and that includes my daughter. So I guess the bastard's going to get away with it. I still let him know I'll never forget it every chance I get. Would you believe he tells his friends I'm sick—that I just hallucinate wildly and that's his burden to bear? He's always ready for me to expose what he did to me—it's like he's turning the whole town against me! They view me as the crazy woman. I just whisper to him, 'You're goin' to hell you know 'cause you can't bullshit God.' "

Melissa's father called me to tell me that he felt sorry for her. He attributed her claims of rape or abuse to somebody else or to her imagination. He launched quite a campaign on the phone that day to exonerate himself. Yet he did not convince me. When she was an adolescent, Melissa had the typical profile of someone abused as a child: she was an alcoholic at thirteen, sexually promiscuous throughout her teens, had some involvement with drugs, and generally projected a defiantly seductive image. Melissa's descriptions of the events involving her father were consistent, including his presence in the house when no one was home, the physical details of his body, and his characteristic ways of doing things. In addition, he had brutally beaten her when she was younger, throwing her down a flight of stairs. His other two daughters verified to me his brutality toward Melissa and to no one else in the family, because they had witnessed it. For all these reasons, I believe her claims of rape and physical abuse at his hands.

Melissa's treatment involved an intense use of interpretation of her transference to me. She was struggling to structure the relationship between therapist and patient to resemble and perpetuate the relationship between herself and her father, just as she had done with other boys and men. Outwardly it appeared she behaved this way because she could not hope for anything better. But Melissa had two reasons for this posture, neither of them conscious: one was to perpetuate the early experience with her father because that was familiar; the other was to prove to herself that she could both "take it" (being raped) but also—this time, with other men—take charge of the sex. In psychoanalytic theory this drive to repeat a negative experience with the wish to change the outcome, usually in a way that would restore a sense of control to a person who had been made to feel helpless, is referred to as a *repetition compulsion*. Melissa repeated her trauma in a way that made her feel powerful through sexual attractiveness. Giving up this role with men meant feeling powerless again. As her therapist I was asking her to relinquish this defense, even though I understood its value to her and knew she would find it difficult to do.

The pitfalls of winning the Oedipal romance   Therapy with a compulsively seductive patient poses many extraordinary challenges, the first of which is how confrontational the situation is for both parties. The transference can be so intense that the patient may terminate the therapy. To keep the situation under control, the therapist must continually and carefully ask, what is happening between the two people in the room. This allows the interpretation of transference to remain an ongoing process—as both a reassurance and clarification for the patient, and a reminder to the therapist to maintain good boundaries.

Without this check, the therapeutic process could break down. The worst outcome would be for the patient to succeed in seducing her therapist sexually. Indeed, civil court records and professional discipline hearings are replete with such irresponsible and unethical errors in judgment by therapists, who were justly punished for their actions. Sexual behavior between therapist and patient does additional damage to the patient because she will experience it as a reenactment of the original abuse.

Complicating father-daughter incest is *the Oedipal romance*, which is universal and healthy in childhood development: A young daughter depends on her father for protection, guidance, and her sense of femininity. At the same time she experiences feelings toward her father that we term Oedipal: he is her hero. Between ages three to six she is likely to go through a time when she thinks she is "in love" with daddy and may even announce to others that she plans to marry him when she grows up. These feelings are the beginnings of what will evolve into her desire for future heterosexual romance with boys and other men as she matures. The Oedipal romance referred to here is an innocent affection, devoid of actual sexual acts. When sexual acts between father and daughter do take place, all sense of protection and self-worth vanishes.

The therapeutic relationship between a male therapist and a female patient invites the transference of these natural childhood feelings between daughter and father. When the therapist allows the relationship to become sexualized, he is repeating the violation of the natural healthy bond, putting the patient into a state of dependent despair and verifying her feelings that all men will use her sexually for their own pleasure, disregarding her value as a person.

Ideally every therapist, regardless of gender, strives to interpret the behavior and language of his or her patient always keeping the patient's welfare the highest priority. Psychotherapy, sometimes thought more an art than a science, requires a delicate endeavor to balance real caring with important professional boundaries. Like any human endeavor it is never perfect—but it is often successful. This success belongs to both the therapist and the patient.

28

Tasks and Challenges Facing the Therapist

Most beginning therapists have two major fears: damaging the patient by saying the "wrong" thing—something that might be construed as hurtful or insensitive by the patient—or sounding inadequate or uninteresting to the patient, causing her to leave therapy. When the reason for therapy is childhood sexual abuse, additional issues confront the therapist. He or she may be transported back to those early work years, when he or she was filled with self-doubt, offered too many uncontrolled expressions of sympathy, and generally had a sense of inadequacy. As the therapist acquires more skill and experience—which can only come with time and study—these fears lessen.

A good starting point for both is a mutually agreed-upon list of goals for the treatment. In addition to articulating goals, it is often helpful for the therapist to describe the conflicts likely to arise between patient and therapist and to emphasize to the patient that these conflicts are part of therapy and should not be a cause for either party to terminate treatment.

"ONE FOOT OUT THE DOOR"

Despite the best of plans and explanations made earlier in therapy, feelings can arise that risk sabotaging therapeutic goals and resolutions. Patients who make the therapist feel like he or she is "walking on eggshells" threaten to render the therapist useless if the therapist is being *too* careful of the patient's feelings. Katie was such a patient. Katie was so sensitive that a wrong word by a therapist could cause her to lose faith in both the person and the therapeutic process. She would harbor grievances during sessions and days later e-mail me or leave voicemail messages about the ways I had been destructive to her sense of trust.

After explaining my statements in response to two complaints, I realized that her intent was to keep me on the defensive. My sympathy for her brutal past had clouded my awareness of the dynamic that was transpiring between us. After receiving the next e-mail with its not-so-veiled accusation, I responded, "Are you collecting grievances?"

She answered, "I guess I'm grouchy and trying to be a smart-ass."

We had broken through an aspect of transference I call "one foot out the door," a resistant patient's ever-present willingness to quit therapy. I was then freer to confront her about the way this behavior, which she did not limit to me, affected her other relationships as well. Katie had lost several recent friendships as a result of her tendency to put people on the defensive and make them feel guilty. In earlier sessions she recounted her hurt feelings over these incidents, apparently unaware that she had driven the friends away. Discussing these situations in those sessions had helped her understand her impact on other people. But the real turning point came when she was confronted with the same dynamic in her behavior toward me. Katie's therapy then moved ahead, free of her constant implicit threat to terminate.

SUSTAINING THERAPY OVER THE LONG TERM

Many of the comments to follow repeat points made in other chapters, but the ability to sustain a helpful therapeutic relationship over a period of many years is so critical to the patient's recovery that it behooves us to emphasize them again. Survivors of child sexual abuse suffer a lot, and medication assists by providing the patient relief from some of that suffering. In addition, medication also helps to expedite therapy, and an intense, consistent therapeutic relationship over time is what will diminish the patient's suffering in the long term. Because this relationship allows the patient to develop emotional vulnerability, therapy provides an open window to change, as well as the potential to improve the patient's expectations of the kinds of relationships she could have with others.

For the psychotherapist, sustaining a consistent, long-term therapeutic relationship is a tall order—made taller when the patient has other difficulties. These may include negative current living situations (such as ongoing destructive relationships with family members), divorce, or abuse of alcohol or drugs by the patient or people close to her. The first stage of treatment, as emphasized earlier, consists of the therapist's fostering the development of the patient's trust in the process and, of course, in the therapist. This trust then evolves into dependency and attachment. Since she has likely come to therapy with a weak or nonexistent ability to be dependent and form attachments, she will feel at first as if she is granting someone an invitation to mistreat her again. Nevertheless, it is likely that when these aspects of the therapeutic relationship develop, positive change will occur.

Treating patients with childhood sexual abuse in their background demands confidence and comfort on the part of the therapist because of the complex and challenging nature of the delicate therapeutic relationship required. It is also rarely appropriate to treat this type of patient if the therapist is inexperienced. With any patient, establishing trust, dependency, and attachment can pose problems for the therapist, but this is especially true for this group. It is not easy for the survivor to allow someone to take on the role of an authority figure who is also truly helpful because it requires giving up the protection of her current defenses. It is like asking her to take down her "fences" (defenses), which protect her from wild animals (flashbacks and further abuse) in the hope that a protective being or beings can and will replace these fences.

Other therapists have asked me, "How do your patients ever leave you or outgrow their need for you?" Yet when we therapists are effective, patients do outgrow their need for us and eventually do leave. Therapy is a process with a beginning, a middle, and an end. No matter how intense the patient's feelings are for the therapist during the first phase of treatment, this intensity weakens as she gradually becomes an individual with more coping skills, including a better ability to trust and relate to others. Finally she reaches a point when she has replaced the therapist—as an object of trust, attachment, and dependency—with other people whom she has allowed to become close and significant to her in many ways. Then therapy is finished and the patient terminates. Chapter 29 delves into the challenges of pacing therapy.

PROVIDING AN INTERPERSONAL THERAPEUTIC RELATIONSHIP

As we noted in Chapter 27, the therapist has to give him- or herself permission to genuinely care about these patients. Therapy needs to be professional—limited by boundaries—and yet it must also be real in terms of caring. Reacting appropriately to patients' sensitivity (stemming from their sad and traumatic childhood) is dependent on the therapist's ability to make decisions about what kind of responses will be helpful, strengthening their self-esteem and compensating for the negative messages they have received from others. This requires the therapist to have a large repertoire of approaches because he or she must react to a wide variety of personalities in patients who have been affected in different ways by their early experiences. We have seen examples of this diversity among June, Gina, Kendra, Rose, Cassie, Jen, and Maureen.

The therapist also needs to be comfortable in the presence of the patient's pain so the patient can allow it to emerge in sessions.

The therapist must also learn to gently confront the patient when necessary. Some of these abilities can be learned; others are qualities that are either part of the therapist's nature or not.

Because the damage of childhood sexual abuse is caused by an injurious interpersonal relationship, this trauma and all that accompanies it derive from the interpersonal. (We will parse the interpersonal aspects of therapy in more detail in Chapter 31.) No treatment, no matter what its theoretical base or techniques can be complete in assisting recovery without an interpersonal relationship that counters the negative effects of, and can make up for, the original malignant relationship that set the patient's dysfunction in motion. The therapeutic relationship must either rebuild the survivor's lost trust or build new trust where it never existed.

The assumption here is that within each of us there exists a desire to have another person in our lives whom we can trust and depend on for emotional support and protection. This desire may be suppressed within the survivor in order for her to adequately function in the world, allowing her to get through each day without consciously feeling terror, loneliness, or vulnerability to harm by others.

Establishing a relationship that aids the patient in reorganizing her sense of safety—which has been stunted for so long by the traumatic abuse is no small task for her would-be helper. It will take a long time for her brain's characteristic responses to internal associations and external stimuli to change. The helper, in most cases a therapist, has to use the therapeutic relationship to gently and consistently create enough security to change the defenses in the patient's mind and the altered biology of the brain.

This may sound more like a job for a brain surgeon—assisting the hippocampus to literally grow larger and diffusing traumatic material from the amygdala—but, unlike a computer, in which the software cannot change its hardware, the "software" of the mind *can* change some of the "hardware" of the brain. Since one person has created the trauma, another is required to remove it with the tools of the interpersonal relationship. Unfortunately, just as an explosive destroys in an instant a structure that took years to build and will require years to rebuild, it takes years to remove the explosive results of trauma caused by childhood sexual abuse. The mind and brain need time to test for potential harm and allay suspicions of betrayal before reorganization can begin. It is as if mind and brain are saying, "Never again!" The survivor's faith will be slow in coming.

Earlier we mentioned that survivors of childhood sexual abuse usually come to treatment with other presenting problems—primarily behavioral disorders, such as self-mutilation and to a lesser extent eating disorders. Perhaps this is a way for the patient to unconsciously test the treatment, by trying it out on a more tangible, "external" problem. If the therapist demonstrates trustworthiness with this overt issue, the patient's unconscious will allow deeper issues, including those around childhood abuse to emerge. In the first stage of treatment she gives the therapist time to prove trustworthiness and effectiveness. As the intensity of her trust, of her dependency on him or her, and of her attachment grow, so does her capacity for change. The personality of the therapist must allow for this intensity. It is temporary (or should be), but it is also vital to the process of change.

What is involved in the development and fostering of this intense trust? It is important in the process to talk to the patient in a way that convinces her that she is understood. To do so, the therapist must be thoroughly acquainted with the psychological dynamics of childhood sexual abuse, only then can he or she understand the patient's thoughts and feelings and her reactions to other people. Demonstrating this understanding gives the therapist the needed credentials of empathy and compassion in the patient's mind.

An important part of this "credentialing" process is validating the thoughts, feelings, and ideas of the patient's that go unexpressed. This is especially true with a patient who has difficulty articulating her experiences. She may describe her emotional state simply as a vague, intensely negative feeling. If the abuse occurred early in her cognitive development, she had no way to "think about" the event, either at the time or as she grew into adulthood. Consequently she now lacks the vocabulary to communicate her despair. By helping her learn how to articulate that despair—and other feelings as well—the therapist facilitates the creation of a significant partnership.

In addition to articulating feelings the therapist needs to be comfortable explicitly discussing areas of the body, as well as describing abusive acts when necessary. Patients vary with regard to their need to talk about the details of anatomy and of the abuse, so the therapist should be guided by their readiness for these difficult discussions.

29

Pacing in Therapy

The pace at which the therapist approaches issues and symptoms will vary according to the patient's tolerance for the discussion of sensitive topics. Other aspects also affect pacing: several of which are discussed in this chapter: shyness, family pressure, patient resistance, and the strain on the patient who has never approached the subject of her abuse.

LONG-HELD SECRETS REQUIRE SLOW PACING

Most survivors of childhood sexual abuse have been living with their secrets for many years. Typically, the first time they speak about the abuse is in therapy, having kept it a secret since childhood. The longest period of secret keeping I have encountered is forty-one years. For a survivor with a long history of silence, the pacing in therapy is critically important. The therapist must have patience with the slow pace of disclosure, change, and progress in therapy.

What happens to a person who's psychological and personality development has to evolve while carrying this secret? In Part Two, we saw outcomes in a number of women that involved dramatic and endangering behaviors, self-sabotage, timidity, rage, sexual impairment, sexual aggressiveness, social impairments, self-hatred, self-devaluation, and many other problems. These can be traced step-by-step back to abuse that occurred—and to the results that have been incubating, in some cases, for more than twenty years. This means that as the identity of the young child developed during and after the period of abuse, she had to continually redefine herself—as a five-year-old, a twelve-year-old, a sixteen-year-old, and so on, into adulthood—all the while keeping this toxic secret. It is hard to overestimate the damage occurring during these crucial developmental years. The abused child had to define the events and their meanings with no guidance from another person or persons with a mature perspective. She had to learn to live without help in understanding herself. It is no wonder, then, that her response to the abuse evolved into negative ideas, impairments, and self-destructive "solutions" that profoundly affected every aspect of her life.

It is also no surprise that, in asking for help after so much time has been spent without it, disclosing her secret produces so much anxiety. Another individual's interpretations of her emotional life will seem alien to her. She has had very little experience with accepting another person's input. Even if the interpretations are positive, they may not be welcome. They will be competing with long-held ideas that have formed her personality and given it coherence and meaning. Indeed, fear of losing such coherence can contribute to her resistance to therapy. It is easy to forget that when a therapist urges the patient to change for her own good, she is being asked to give up an integral part of herself.

The early stages of therapy   Pacing during the early stages of therapy has been discussed a number of times earlier in the book, but they bear repeating here. Talking and explaining to a survivor of childhood sexual abuse how the abuse might have affected her is often how the therapist begins to build trust. At first the survivor is reluctant to acknowledge that something valid has been said. A therapist may find him- or herself talking to an outwardly nonresponsive listener. Or the patient may merely report (state without feeling or reliving) episodes of abuse. Because reporting is safer for the patient, it represents a good first step toward coming out of isolation concerning these episodes. Although the survivor is reluctant to acknowledge the credibility of the explanations and descriptions being offered by the therapist about what she has gone through, that does not mean she disbelieves them.

During the early stages of treatment, the therapist may have to do a lot of the talking, without receiving confirmation or validation from the patient that he or she is on the right track. There is some risk of making incorrect interpretations or misreading the patient. When that happens, she may say, "No, that's not it," or frown and shake her head. Knowing he or she is not always right when interpreting an inexpressive patient, the therapist can simply acknowledge that fact ("I see you disagree with what I said") and move on with the session. But when the patient is passive, silent, or nonresponsive, in all likelihood she is trying to find out how wise and sensitive the therapist is about her secrets and the workings of her mind. She simply wants to hear more until she can determine the therapist's trustworthiness.

Once she feels the therapist might be trustworthy, transference begins to develop. Then she will start to behave the way she has with potential predators or other difficult adults in her life. This is an unconscious tactic, her way of resisting having to change her outlook or relinquish her defenses. And this is why the therapist must interpret transference and its accompanying behavior as it arises. The therapist is challenging the patient to *consciously* understand and revise the defense mechanisms she has developed and relied on to get through her trauma and that have made her life bearable since then.

This part of the process takes quite a while, and both therapist and patient must be patient and not pursue this most intense phase of the therapy relentlessly. The pace of therapy must reflect the seriousness of the task. (As mentioned in Chapter 27, however, light moments and even light sessions are needed to prevent the therapy from becoming so painfully heavy that the patient either withdraws from therapy or from discussions of serious issues, causing the talk to become shallow.)

In many cases the initial reason for entering therapy is self-mutilation or some other behavioral disorder. It can take up to a year to treat the presenting "acting out" symptom before it is possible to move on to the transference phase described above. However, attending to any overlying disorders is essential. Part Two includes several case studies that illustrate this; work with Colleen provides another example:

Colleen: A case of very early abuse   At eighteen, Colleen was referred to therapy for cutting, which occurred during bouts of severe depression that lasted for months and were sometimes accompanied by panic attacks. She had made at least one suicide gesture.

Colleen and I made substantial progress in reducing the frequency of her cutting episodes but not the depression or the panic attacks. One day, after a silence of several minutes, she said, "I have these flashbacks."

"Do you want to say what they are?"

She looked away. "I'm in the shower with my father. I'm a year old. He does things to me. He probably thinks because I'm too young to talk I won't be able to remember it. When I begin to learn how to talk, he stops. I think to this day he doesn't believe I remember."

"Do you want to say more about the content of the flashbacks?"

"No. They're fragments. I just know what it felt like—what he did. I don't want to talk about it anymore."

Colleen refused to talk about her father's behavior, but a few weeks later brought up a boyfriend she had at fourteen. "He raped me ten times. I kept count. He said he would kill my whole family if I told anyone. I still see him around my neighborhood. He did all that that to me four years ago. Now he's so weird: everybody thinks that he's crazy, so I just avoid talking to him."

Colleen had started keeping her secrets before she could talk. It was at age one that she learned about violation and the lack of protection available in her world. She had to lower her expectations of her family, friends, and teachers. When her boyfriend raped her at fourteen, she was frightened and in pain, but somewhere inside of her was a memory of violation and the absence of protection. When this teenage boy threatened her with harm to her family, she made a choice to tell no one. She had no experience with protection. She felt she would have to live with unwanted intercourse. More than four years had gone by when she spoke about it to me. She knew that the sex with her boyfriend was actually rape but had never said it out loud before. She had not been ready to name it even to herself when there was no one to tell about it and how it made her feel. In fact, Colleen had never really confided in anyone with regard to her feelings and had not developed communication skills in this area.

Colleen's speaking style and facial expression did not match her subject matter. When she was describing something sad and frightening, she would express herself in a low-key style, sulky and brief, often minimizing or denying the impact of the event. When she was discussing an unemotional event or telling a story about a party, she would speak in a cheery, rapid style. When she was recounting a grievance she had with a professor, her manner would be intense, irate, and indignant. When the topic was about something that had deeply hurt her, she would be somber, yet if asked how she felt about it, she would shrug off its importance. It seemed that Colleen was not accustomed to processing her feelings before trying to talk about them, a clear sign of emotional repression.

She had kept her first secret for 95 percent of her life. It was as if a child molested at five told her story for the first time at the age of eighty. That is a long time to keep a secret. It would take a long time for her to gradually express her outrage and be able to understand all the ways the abuse had affected her personality and character. Along with self-understanding would come a more authentic way of expressing her feelings, both to herself and to others. Progress would be gradual so Colleen and I would have to commit to the long haul. With a patient who has kept her secrets a very long time, as Colleen had, it is important to explain early in treatment that recovery will be slow, so that the patient, as well as her therapist, can maintain that perspective.

PRESSURE FROM THE FAMILY

Upon beginning therapy for childhood sexual abuse, it is important to differentiate between the different kinds of abuses because they affect the victim in different ways. Recall from Chapter 20 that the relationships between the victim and the perpetrator, the varied behavioral ways the abuses were committed, and the frequency of these episodes all affect the developing personality in different ways from childhood through adolescence and finally to adulthood. This information enables us to take the mystery out of the "strangeness" that both survivors and those close to them experience.

A serious threat to proper pacing in therapy is pressure from the family to produce quick results in terms of the patient's relief from symptoms. Parents or other family members may call the therapist asking, "When will the cutting [or other detectable symptoms] stop?" Family members may lose sight of the fact that it takes a long time to recover from childhood sexual abuse and that, until substantial progress is made in therapy, coexisting symptoms of any disorders the patient has will continue.

The family's impatience is likely to affect the patient, especially if the parents express frustration with their daughter over what she is doing to herself and berate her to stop. Ironically, this may drive her deeper into her symptoms, cause her to shut down emotionally, and reverse the progress she has made in developing the extraordinary trust she is working toward in therapy. In emotional terms, this pressure just reaffirms what her first perpetrator demonstrated—that there is no protection for her. Her family's complaints also suggest to her that her therapist cannot protect her from being judged inadequate by others, taking her back to her own feelings of worthlessness caused by her abuse. The therapist must inform the significant people in the patient's life, such as parents and teachers, that damage from child abuse takes years to repair, and that if they have questions they should call the therapist instead of berating the patient.

Some families go so far as to make treatment conditional, suggesting they will stop paying for the therapy if they do not see marked improvement in symptoms by a certain time. When the patient is threatened with cancellation of therapy, she immediately protects herself by withdrawing her trust for the therapist, fearing that he or she may soon be taken away from her. This may be a good time to invite the family in for a session so that they can witness the progress the patient has made in other areas, such as communication.

This is not an issue for patients who are legally adult and self-supporting, but it affects teenagers and those adult patients who are dependent on their parents for financial support.

PACING WITH A SHY PATIENT

The child's mind observes every lesson it is taught. It reacts by structuring that child's personality growth for protection from harm, fear, and pain. In so doing, the general personality characteristics of the child are formed. When we meet teenage girls who are troubled, they may seem shy, withdrawn, or impulsive. In fact, they are taking defensive measures to avoid getting hurt. What we are seeing in their demeanor is their anticipation of being frightened or hurt by others.

This kind of girl reacts by pushing other people away with behaviors that intimidate, worry, or let others know that she demands extraordinary distance. She is not open about herself: she does not get close or personal in discussions, even though she can be outgoing, and even cheerful, during a fun group activity. It is that underlying barrier to closeness in social, romantic, or even school and work activities that others come up against when they occasionally try to engage her in a personal conversation.

We have all heard the expression, "She's a private person." Most of the time we just accept that, but do we ever wonder why she requires more privacy than the rest of us? I am not suggesting that on a social level we ought to confront her by invading her privacy, even if we feel rejected by her distancing behavior. Shy people are uncomfortable with closeness but are often mistaken for being snobs. This is how so many abused girls go unnoticed.

A therapist treating someone whose shyness has become integral to her personality must pace the therapy accordingly. Understanding that she lacks the ability to express herself, the therapist can begin by talking for her. The therapist does this by making statements about how the patient might be feeling, then asking the patient if these statements ring true. The patient need only say yes or no. In this way she begins to converse about her feelings in a minimal way. In the next step, the therapist continues talking empathically but now asks the patient to "chime in" with sentence-length comments. Multiple-choice questions about her feelings can also be helpful in encouraging her to speak. In this way she gradually gets used to conversing. Over time her shyness lessens and she begins to initiate talk.

CHALLENGING THE PATIENT

Until now in this chapter, we have been discussing ways to keep the pacing of therapy slow and measured, which is necessary for patients recovering from childhood sexual abuse. Occasionally, however, the pacing needs to be stepped up, as when sessions appear to be going nowhere: The patient may be having difficulty in disclosing pain, showing her feelings, or being expressive in her talking style. She is probably afraid of becoming close to the therapist because of her characteristic discomfort with closeness. Then it may be appropriate to challenge her, not simply wait her out.

For example, one way a patient can stall therapy is by distancing herself with one-word responses, as if to say, "Everything's okay— keep away!" If the therapist starts a session by asking, "How are you?" or "How was your weekend?" she might repeatedly answer, "Fine," or "Nothing new." Eventually the therapist runs out of questions. This impasse may be a good time for a silence until she can come up with her own agenda for conversation. Or the thera- pist can assist her with self-expression by reading her body lan- guage and expressing it verbally, as I had to do with Jen.

Some days Jen came in with lots to talk about, usually events in her life. On other days, when she was struggling with emotional questions and conflicts, she would fuss with items in her bag, books, or her cell phone despite the sign on my door that reads, Please Turn Off Cell Phones. The way Jen would fuss indicated she was in conflict: it was deliberate, intense, and silent; her face was set in a perplexed look, and she made no eye contact with me. On those days I would not ask her the usual small talk questions to get started but instead would ask her directly what the problem was. Here is what transpired in one such interchange:

"What's the matter?"

"Nothing," Jen replied, "Why do you ask?"

"Your face is set. You aren't making eye contact, and won't even give me a polite greeting. That means something is wrong."

She fussed a bit more and said, "Do you think I'm crazy?"

"What happened today to make you ask that question?"

She slumped down in the overstuffed chair, relaxed her muscles, waved her arms about and shook her head. "I lost it today in school. The teacher was talking, and I started banging on my books and repeatedly shouting, 'You're wrong!' until everyone in the class was looking at me. The teacher just looked at me and said, 'Jen, are you all right?' The other students looked a little rattled. One kid repeated, 'Are you okay?' Somebody else asked, 'Is there anything wrong?' Apparently I was also crying, but I didn't notice it. I just put my head down until it passed. Everybody was good about it, and the class continued so I wouldn't be embarrassed. I'm glad I go to a smart college. Nobody brought it up until the class ended and the teacher came up to me and asked, 'Will you be all right to go home?' I said, "Yeah, I'm going to my therapist's office from here.' He nodded and said, 'Good.' So now that I told you what happened, do you think I'm crazy?"

"That's a pretty harsh label. Something might have set you off. Do you have any idea what that would be?"

"No. I wasn't thinking about anything. It just happened." She became teary. "So what kind of a brain do I have? That's not normal."

"No, that's not normal, and yes, you lost it, and for a while there you experienced confused thought and energy that sounded angry."

"But I had no reason to be angry. Isn't that crazy?"

"Jen, once in a while this will happen. It will become less frequent and less intense until finally it's gone. It's understandable that after something like this happens you feel demoralized and 'crazy.' You are recovering. It's better now than it was two years ago or last year. Maybe in another year these episodes will be gone. But that doesn't mean you won't lose your temper—though it will be with realistic provocation, instead of randomly like today."

"So I'll be crazy until next year?"

"You're not crazy. You have episodes of confusion, and they go away within two hours. After that, you're okay and understandably upset about the episode. We'll keep working until they gradually disappear. 'Gradually' means each month you'll be better."

"I wish I didn't have this in the first place." She wiped her eyes and sighed.

Due to her embarrassment and fear of "being crazy," Jen might not have mentioned the classroom incident or shared her anxiety if instead I had begun this session by asking, "How are you?" and I had accepted the inevitable brief reply at face value. Patients with similar problems or histories often need this kind of help in disclosing their painful self-doubts.

Jen's episodes of "losing it" did diminish and go away over the next year, though it would be some time before she would trust her mind not to become chaotic or produce periods of amnesia. Jen also took medication to minimize the episodes and the plan was for her to stay medicated for an indefinite period of time. As the interval between episodes lengthened, the likelihood of the next episode occurring kept diminishing. Pacing therapy with Jen meant allowing for her uneven moods in sessions and directing her gently out of them until she was more stable and appropriate in her responses. She also needed mild confrontations when she became unresponsive; it usually meant something was worrying her, as in the session just recounted.

When we began therapy, Jen's communication took the form of shouting at me as if I were the person or situation that had offended her. I understood that this behavior was a combination of dissociation and distancing from therapy; I also knew she was not ready to have me interpret this to her. As treatment progressed over two years, she improved enough for me to be able to challenge her on her manner of speaking to me: "Why are you shouting at me? I am not being offensive toward you."

"I'm just nervous—I didn't mean to be shouting at you."

Jen's ability to accept a "reality check" in session and to own her feeling of nervousness indicated a big improvement in her coping ability. This was a radical change from her first year of treatment when I would have gotten a combative response from her. Had I challenged her at that time, it would have caused her to maintain her distance and to see me as being indistinguishable from other people who might scare or harm her, especially strangers. The process of therapy was decreasing the chaotic ways her amygdala worked (which were causing confusion and producing dissociative states) and increasing the strength of her hippocampus (which prevented dissociation and helped her make more orderly distinctions). As a result, Jen began to see me as someone who was not likely to hurt her. To use the analogy offered in Chapter 28, Jen is a classic example of a person's "software" adjusting her "hardware," and it all hinged on properly pacing her therapy, not rushing her during this intense part of the process, but also not being afraid to confront her at appropriate times.

When the pace of therapy best matches the patient's ability to cope with the stress of exploring her history and her feelings about that history, the most progress will be made. Trial and error at the start of each patient's therapy is inevitable. This chapter has touched on several stumbling blocks to proper pacing, but if the therapy is to be successful, the trial-and-error phase must evolve into an effective working relationship.

30

Repairing the Damage:
Reducing the Effects of Trauma

A s emphasized earlier, trauma is such a powerful shock to the brain that the psychotherapist who works with a trauma survivor is competing not only with the psychological effects of the experience but with strong neurobiological defenses as well. Activation of these defenses continually occurs despite the best efforts of therapist and patient, and it happens at seemingly lightning speed. These neurological impulses are responsible for such phenomena as flashbacks, dissociation, amnesia, and blurred thinking in general.

COMBINING PSYCHOTHERAPY WITH MEDICATION

Medication is usually required—at least temporarily—to compensate the survivor's brain chemically for what the trauma did to it. Medication works by reducing the random neurological impulses that interrupt the continuity of thoughts and feelings and thereby interfere with therapy-induced change. The last section of this chapter discusses selective appropriate medication.

Nevertheless, medication is only valuable in removing the neurological roadblocks. To move forward toward the goal of strengthening the cortex (the center of conscious thought, reflection, and decision making in the brain) and the hippocampus (the seat of orderly memory the brain's limbic system) requires the "engine" of therapy. By developing and combining a trusting relationship with the patient to revise ideas and to develop new perspectives, therapy effectively strengthens the more organized and "reasonable" cortex to override "unreasonable" messages from the amygdala.

Religious conviction, hypnosis, and biofeedback might be alternative methods. However, the likelihood of any of these approaches successfully competing with the neurological effects of trauma on the amygdala is slim without medication. On the other hand, a well-coordinated combination with medication, psychotherapy, and perhaps one or more alternative methods should prove helpful.

As discussed in earlier chapters, the first goal of the therapist is to help the patient accept the therapist as a safe person, someone she does not need to distance herself from. The first phase of treatment could last from a few months to a year or longer. When both therapist and patient can accept confrontation and can interpret their relationship—without trauma-related reactions from the patient—the process of diminishing trauma can begin in earnest: the patient can now use her therapeutic alliance with the therapist to begin to reverse the effects created by her abuser, who created the trauma.

The assumption here is that when the abuse-induced trauma was caused by one person, creating a damaging psychological reaction in the survivor, another person, through a therapeutic relationship, can reverse much of that damage. Unfortunately, as mentioned earlier the reversal takes much longer than the initial trauma-inducing experience. Part of this process requires both emotional and biological recovery. Regarding the latter, researchers have found that rats subjected to electric shock only once, on their way to obtaining food, require one hundred and twelve trials before they abandon evasive and halting behavior when pursuing food in that setting.[8] This is a natural biological response. And although people are not rats, both humans and rats are mammals, and thus neurologically we humans are very similar to rats. Such research is important for aiding the therapeutic community to make appropriate applications of medication and behavioral therapy when we strive for recovery. It also helps to explain why the time needed for recovery is proportional to the length of time that has elapsed since the traumatic events occurred.

Conversations in the second phase of therapy are freer now that trust in the therapeutic alliance has been established. At this stage, the therapist is free to be more direct about what is happening in the room between therapist and patient. The patient has the same increased freedom, now that she is not afraid of "saying the wrong thing." At the beginning her fear of therapy was as intense as her fear of being abused. Now it has been reduced to a level of ordinary disagreement.

ROSE: HEALING FROM PROFOUND TRAUMA

Rose (Chapter 9) was a patient whose memories of traumatic sexual abuse (being repeatedly raped by her uncle, who was also her babysitter) were repressed throughout childhood and adolescence. They emerged suddenly in young adulthood when she decided to lose what she believed to be her virginity. Her sudden recollection of the abuse was so intense, including psychotic episodes, that the initial effects of the trauma had to be reduced by focusing discussion on the "new" memories. These were difficult and tearful conversations for her.

Rose had experienced such a severe level of trauma that, like Jen, as an adult she suffered from episodes of dissociative amnesia disorder. Her flashbacks in therapy were filled with expressive terror (screaming and crying) and graphic descriptions of blood flowing from her vagina (". . . as if it was pouring out").

It is important to note here that once Rose remembered the abuse we needed to "shift gears" in her therapy. Though at first she had felt safe and comfortable with a male therapist, she now had to renegotiate the first phase of therapy—establishing trust.

Despite medications to lessen the intensity of remembering her trauma, Rose frequently lapsed into different manners of speech, sometimes sounding trancelike. In one instance she accused me of being "one of them." When I asked, "One of whom?" she responded with, "Men. You're a man. I can't trust a man about anything."

"You can't trust me because I might assault you?"

"Yes, any of you might."

"I understand you feeling that way."

Her trancelike gaze was fixed on the carpet. To bring her back to the here and now, I put my hand out in the line of her gaze, then slowly moved my hand to my face. Her eyes followed my hand until she was looking at me.

"I think you just dissociated—are you back now?"

With that she came out of the trance, and resumed her normal tone and cadence of speech. "I guess I should trust you, though. You encouraged me to enroll in that self-defense course." Then pointing her index finger at me she said, "I could protect myself from you." She was gradually bringing herself into her present, realistic state of security.

"What provoked you to dissociate today? Did someone frighten you?"

"No, sometimes I just 'go there' when I need to feel safe. It happens if I spend too much time with my parents—who invited him to rape me!" she exclaimed, referring to the fact that her parents had left her alone with her live-in uncle. "I have to feel safe. Sometimes when I'm very anxious, I think that they could invite someone else to do the same thing to me even though I know I'm grown up and have my own apartment. I fear the past can recur, even though logically I know they wouldn't do it. It's like, just being around them reminds me of the whole thing and makes me feel helpless. And I dissociate. Will that ever go away?"

"It will take a long time. Today you came out of it quickly with only a hint from me. We have established some 'dissociation breakers' already. It's been a year, but you kept your secret for nearly ten years."

"So I'm going to be a lot of trouble for you for a long time."

"Probably, but not as much trouble as you are to yourself."

"Will that make you hate me?"

"No, but I will feel sorry for you when you're in pain."

"If I'm not in pain will you get bored with me?"

"I think you're trying to figure out all the possible ways therapy and our relationship might go wrong. It only can go wrong if you stop coming in before we're done working on this."

"You won't tell me to stop coming here?"

"No. You, or we, will decide when you should stop coming, and that will be a long time from now. We have your problem with dissociation to work on, and after that we have a long list of 'missing pieces' to fill in and repairs to make."

"Are you sure you won't get sick of me?"

"I won't even get sick of reassuring you."

"Okay, I get the point."

It took Rose years to recover from her trauma and the dissociations, flashbacks, amnesias, and panic attacks resulting from it. As we continued to reestablish trust we not only could talk about what she was going through; she could also become demanding and challenging in our sessions. This made her feel more secure and diminished the power of chaotic memories that assaulted her. It wasn't one dramatic or clever session that changed everything for the better, but rather the ongoing reliability of the therapeutic relationship, full of give-and-take, which brought Rose further from the trauma-inducing relationship and experiences with which she came to therapy.

SELECTING MEDICATION

Critical to success in using the model suggested here (psychotherapy combined with medication) are the skills and experience not only of the psychotherapist in working with trauma patients, but also of the psychiatrist in making the best choice of medication.

When making the decision to put a patient on psychiatric medication, the first question the psychiatrist asks is, What effects do we want the medication to have? Answering this question requires diagnosing and defining all the conditions and disorders the patient is suffering from. The patient's moods, impulses, anxieties, thought patterns, behavior patterns, and general emotional and mental discomfort have to be taken into consideration. Later in this section we take a brief look at the drugs and groups of drugs appropriate for different disorders.

After determining the kinds of effects desired to help the patient, there are further questions to answer: If several drugs are possible candidates, which one is likely to be the best choice? What order should the candidate drugs be tried in, and for how long before concluding that it may be time to dry another drug? What is the best dosage for each drug? Should two or more drugs be combined for best effect? What are the side effects? (All drugs have them.) Unfortunately, medication often has to be chosen by trial and error, since each patient reacts differently to each drug. An experienced psychiatrist will shorten this period of experimentation as much as possible.

Once the medication has been decided on, other issues come into play: How long should the patient stay on each drug? Most of these medications (and others not mentioned in this chapter) may be used either temporarily or long-term (including possibly for the rest of the patient's life). Because of the complexity of using psychotropic medication, the responsibilities of the psychiatrist continue after prescription; for as long as the patient is taking medication, she needs to have regular check-ins with her psychiatrist, who can monitor her for changes in symptoms and side effects, adjust dosages, and change medication where necessary.

Severe anxiety accompanied by impulsivity and dissociation

Lessening these symptoms usually requires medication from the category of *major tranquilizers*, of which there is a lengthy list. In large doses, these act as antipsychotics. The most popularly prescribed drugs in this group presently are Seroquel (quetiapine), Risperdal (risperidone), and Zyprexa (olanzapine), among others.

Depression   The most frequently prescribed group of antidepressants is the *specific serotonin reuptake inhibitors* (SSRIs), which allow the brain to use its own supply of serotonin better; problems with serotonin are a major contributing factor to depression. Often-prescribed SSRIs include Prozac (fluoxetine), Zoloft (sertraline), Paxil (paroxetine), Celexa (citalopram), and Lexapro (escitalopram). Others will be probably be developed in the future, as the search for effective antidepressant medication with the least possible side effects continues.

Bipolar disorder   This is the new term for manic depression. Bipolar disorder is characterized by severe mood swings from extreme highs of the manic phase (grandiosity, rapid speech, and irritability) to extreme lows of the depression phase (profound sadness, immobility, and pessimism). The most often prescribed medications for this disorder are Lamictal (lamotrigene), Topamax (topiramate), Neurontin (gabapentin), and lithium.

Obsessive-compulsive disorders (OCD)   Symptoms of this disorder vary and include the compulsion to endlessly repeat activities and thoughts, even though no positive gains or consequences realistically result from this behavior. For some OCD patients, the focus is contamination fears, which compel them to clean themselves endlessly—far beyond what is reasonable. Medications most commonly prescribed for OCD are Anafranil (clomipramine), and many of the SSRIs mentioned earlier.

General anxiety disorders   Sometimes accompanied by panic attacks, general anxiety disorder often requires medications in the benzodiazepine group, which are used exclusively for this disorder. The list is very long. Most popular of these are Klonopin (clonazepam), Valium (diazepam), Ativan (lorazepam), Librium (chlordiazepoxide), and Xanax (alprazolam). Since the drugs in this group are often abused and can become addictive, psychiatrists are understandably wary when prescribing them.

The latest studies indicate that the highest improvement rate for moderate to severe mental disorders results from the combined used of medication and psychotherapy. It is important that both practitioners collaborate and frequently confer in the treatment of the patient.

31

Taking a Closer Look
at Psychotherapy

Much of the information in this chapter has been presented in different ways in earlier chapters. Here we look at psychotherapy in greater detail. Five aspects of therapy are important for recovery from childhood sexual abuse. Some of them come into play throughout the therapeutic process, while others are prominent during different phases of recovery. First we briefly describe each aspect; then we review two patients profiled earlier in the book to show how differently these aspects can play out in particular cases.

ESTABLISHING THE THERAPIST'S CREDENTIALS FOR TRUSTWORTHINESS

The patient must be able to experience the therapist as reliable and dependable. Character traits such as wisdom, patience, sensitivity, empathy, sincerity, and interest in the patient's recovery comprise much of what the patient needs in the therapist. Additionally, it should be clear that the therapist's personal needs should play no role whatsoever in the treatment relationship.

The therapist must demonstrate knowledge of the area of

patient needs, helping her to form a therapeutic alliance. A successful alliance reduces her need to protect herself from the therapist, which would produce resistance to treatment and recovery. Developing this alliance takes quite a while; often more than a year is needed for the patient to recognize an ally in even the most suitable therapist. For many years the patient has used mistrust, suspicion, and expectations of disappointment as protection against potential abuse by others. This emotional pattern is hard to overcome, even in a motivated patient.

FOSTERING THE PATIENT'S SENSE OF SAFETY

The safest therapeutic environment for a patient is one in which her needs are the clear focus. This means that the therapist will listen carefully and remember what the patient talks about from week to week. He or she must have the skill to elicit the patient's real feelings, no matter how painful, and to stay with the topic at hand without rushing away to a more "comfortable" one. The therapist will demonstrate patience and understanding of negative comments or silence, and try to help the patient achieve insights about her own behavior. The therapist must be reliable and consistent through all phases of treatment—even when the patient is experiencing emotional difficulty that produces erratic progress. In this nonjudgmental environment, trust will develop.

TESTING THE SAFETY OF THE THERAPEUTIC ENVIRONMENT

Following the development of the patient's confidence to "test and act out," the therapist can analyze the talk and challenge her motivation at any given point in the session. This next step may still take some time, as she may have to get comfortable with her newfound freedom in therapy. She needs to find out first that she will not be abandoned, condemned, or disliked. She may fear that she'll make the therapist angry or defensive, weakening him (or her), by acting difficult. When she has had sufficient time to develop faith in the therapist for "passing the test," the therapist may work to facilitate change in the patient's negative self-image or self-destructive behavior by doing some challenging of his or her own.

USING SAFETY TO CREATE CHANGE

The goal of analyzing and challenging the patient's behavior toward the therapist is to help her distinguish actual perpetrators from the rest of the world. Challenging and being challenged in therapy sessions creates a sheltered "workshop" for the patient, where she can experiment with changing her emotional stance toward another person without dangerous consequences.

FORMING A BASIS FOR SELF-TRUST

Developing the patient's comfort in questioning herself starts to break down her feeling that it is her against the rest of the world. She begins to work on "belonging in society." This is a major part of the therapy, since it is her development and solidification of real connections to others that compete with flashbacks and the need to dissociate. The therapy sessions serve as the model for interactions she could have in the world outside of her sessions.

TWO EXAMPLES

Therapy will vary for different patients; despite what they may have in common, each patient is an individual. Colleen and Kendra, both abuse victims, required careful pacing in their respective therapies so that each could approach change in her own way.

Colleen   Colleen (Chapter 29) took nearly a year to tell me about her flashbacks, the abuse she endured as an infant, and the rapes she suffered at the age of fourteen. Since the first time she was violated was so early in her life, she needed a long time to test me before she would trust me. Her therapy progressed at a different pace than it would for someone whose abuse began at a later age. In her case, we had to deal with her cutting, dissociative states, panic attacks, erratic behavior in school, and sessions where she said very little, before I could expect her to volunteer—or even remember—the flashbacks in sessions. She would halt the process by saying, "I don't want to talk about this anymore."

Had Colleen told me about her flashbacks before she was ready, they would have destabilized her and risked exacerbating her other symptoms, which were already improving. In fact, she did some backsliding after several sessions of discussing the abuse. But after a few months her moods were more stable and she was doing better with friends and coping with school, which had previously been a problem. It was still a long time before our sessions allowed for the emotional safety and self-trust sufficient for Colleen to experience the five phases listed above. Then she was able to initiate or tolerate questioning her own motives, actions, and ideas with me in a dialogue.

Kendra   In Kendra's case (Chapter 16) it was her cousins who playfully cajoled her into submitting to being violated by them. At one point she convinced herself that it was normal. It was when she disclosed these "games" to her friends, who then ostracized her, that shame set in.

It was difficult to determine whether the elements of trauma had developed in Kendra. She displayed none of the symptoms. She was comfortable nearly from the first session explicitly disclosing the sequence of events between herself and each of her two cousins. However, the matter-of-fact way she described the details of their behaviors disguised her past and present shame about their sexual interactions. She channeled this shame into compulsively aggressive sexual behavior with young men and suffered from bulimia.

Like many bulimics, Kendra needed to be asked regularly about her eating disorders; if she wasn't, she would try to ignore it. Talking about the symptoms of bingeing and purging brought her painful emotions to the surface, where they could be addressed. To allow this to happen, Kendra first needed to test the safety of therapy. As she developed trust in me and herself, she was able to tolerate having me challenge her symptomatic behavior. The following interchange is an example.

In one session Kendra came in cheerily. I asked her, "How many bulimic episodes have you had this week?"

She responded in an upbeat manner: "Oh, just two or three. I forget."

"You don't seem to be bothered by them."

"Well, I'd rather they didn't happen, but that's life." She shrugged her shoulders.

"Is that real casualness you're portraying to me, or are you trying to keep away from deeper feelings you might have about these episodes?"

"I don't know what you want me to say."

"How do you feel about having binged and stood over a toilet and puked your guts up two or three times this week? It's not a pretty picture."

Kendra looked embarrassed. She protested: "You're supposed to make me feel better. Now I feel disgusting! I feel like everything about me is disgusting! How does that help me?"

"I can't be your enabler. I can't tell you that bingeing is okay, that vomiting to compensate for overeating is okay. I want to help you accept *yourself*, not your sick behavior. I can't say that enticing boys and men to have sex is healthy for you, especially when your motives aren't sexual. When you encounter a male that actually doesn't want to have sex with you but thinks he should want to, so he goes along with it anyway to protect his sense of manhood—that's practically rape on your part. Maybe you haven't realized that your cousins raped you, but your style with men is to castrate them, force them into having sex with you out of shame. You don't know why you're bulimic. You don't know why you conquer men sexually, so you don't have to know you've been humiliated and debased by your cousins. I think you ought to dedicate yourself to finding out who you are— what really makes you feel good and what really doesn't, instead of living symptomatically. You have the right to know when you're ashamed and how to get rid of it and avoid it in the future. You want me to humor you. I don't want therapy to be yet another symptom for you, or another place to hide from yourself. I have more faith in you than that. I think you can emerge healthy."

Kendra stopped crying. "You do?"

"Yes I think you can learn to live without fake sex and fake eating."

"But under it all I do feel filthy. I don't know how you can stand me."

"Maybe I've got a clearer picture of you than you do and can win you over to mine."

"I wish I could believe you."

"That's a good start and we'll need lots of time until you can. Every session you show up for says you're on your way. Gradually you'll get there."

"When will I be better?"

"You're already a little better from what we've dealt with today."

"So I'm not filthy inside?"

"If you can ask, you already have hope."

Kendra was atypical, in that safety in therapy lay in confrontation. She had proved to herself that she could seduce whomever she wanted to, but it left her empty. She needed therapy to help her stop playing the game the world had played with her.

We have taken a look at the struggle that is part of the psychotherapy process. If the patient and therapist emerge with their alliance intact, the most complete recovery is possible.

32

Going Public with Family and Community

How many survivors keep their childhood sexual abuse a secret forever because of the inherent difficulties in disclosure? Certainly it requires great courage to talk about sexual abuse, risking the rejection and disbelief of their community and family.

PUBLIC ATTITUDES AND THEIR EFFECT ON THE SURVIVOR

Because childhood sexual abuse is a painful subject, other people may at first react to disclosure with denial, especially if the abuse involves their loved ones. Moreover, stories and programs in the media frequently portray the survivor's worst fear—that others will react by saying or thinking "She asked for it." Even though this shift of blame from victimizer to victim is generally not leveled at children, people who have been sexually abused, as we have seen repeatedly in this book, blame themselves regardless of how old they were when assaulted.

Perhaps no crime produces more moral outrage than the abuse of children; there is no controversy on this issue. The more difficult issue is addressing events that happened several or many years ago.

The public is uninformed with regard to the kinds of damage that may have occurred in the intervening years since the abuse stopped. Many people assume that the survivor has "gotten over it"—or should have. Now in her late teens or in adulthood, she will not evoke the same sympathetic reaction from others that a recently assaulted distressed child would.

Ironically the damage done to the survivor has only intensified, rather than diminished with the passage of time, which wears down the survivor's spirit. She, too, may feel she is not as sympathetic a victim because of her long silence. As a child she may have doubted whether or not she was to blame. Or, to make sense of these senseless acts, she may have concluded they definitely were her fault. She has carried this feeling through her developmental years and will have to combat it in order to confront her abuser.

A disbelieving community often reinforces the survivor's doubts. When Cassie (Chapter 11) lodged her complaint to friends and neighbors of her parents in the city of her birth, they condemned her for saying such terrible things about a man they had known and respected for years. Denial is a deep-seated part of human nature—a primal defense mechanism; people do not want to believe that bad things can happen, especially at the hands of someone who seems "normal," even "good."

Sometimes the accused abuser actively contributes to the community's disbelief. Melissa (whom we met in Chapter 27) confronted her father about the abuse in the privacy of his home in a small southwestern town. He denied it. Fearing his daughter would go public with her story and damage his standing in his community, he preempted her by telling all the community leaders that his daughter had a mental illness that caused her to hallucinate memories of having been sexually abused by him.

When her father spoke to me, he sounded aggrieved and sad that his daughter would even imagine such things. He hoped that I would talk her out of these strange ideas. (At his first pause I responded by informing him that I would have to tell his daughter that he had called and what was said in the conversation; I also said I would not attempt to influence her ideas about what had transpired between them in her youth.) Melissa, having heard through her sisters about their father's "disinformation campaign," decided not to present her side of the story to their community, since she was sure she would lose the battle for public opinion. Moreover, she worried about the effect it would have on her marriage and family. Instead she chose to withdraw from her relationship with her father, speaking to him only to berate him, and thenceforth allowing her mother but not him to visit her to see her children.

Melissa's story makes understandable why very few women seek vindication from the law or their community and why most will not attempt such a daunting ordeal. In some cases, recovering from the injuries and impairments to mind and body has to happen through a combination of self-validation and self-forgiveness—but no one is capable of these without help. Human nature demands that we use other people to remind us that "we're okay"—that we need not blame ourselves.

One of the tasks of recovery is getting over self-blame. Another task may be planning to confront the abuser and disclose to other family members. Direct confrontation is not always possible, but disclosure to others in the survivor's life usually is. Working with a competent psychotherapist will probably be necessary to help the survivor feel comfortable with disclosure. To enhance recovery, the patient might add a support group. Medication may also be necessary to overcome mental and emotional reactions that her therapeutic and other relationships cannot surmount.

DISCLOSURE WITHIN THE FAMILY

Telling family members is not easy. Depending on family relationships, however, the survivor is often believed, even when the accused perpetrator is the father. Families become divided over this issue and are often never the same. Nevertheless, even if only some members believe her, disclosure allows the survivor to overcome her sense of isolation within her family. Some examples illustrate this:

In Ava's case, (Chapter 14) her mother divorced her father over her disclosures in less than a month after Ava made them.

In Olivia's case (Chapter 12), Olivia and her sisters became estranged from their parents because neither could acknowledge the impact of the abuse: their father denied it completely, while their mother's response indicated she either believed this was a normal part of father-daughter relationships (probably due to the abusive relationship with her own father) or found it more comfortable to excuse, or side with, her wealthy husband. Since Olivia's younger sister took her father to family court over her own abuse, where a convincing case was made on her behalf, Olivia knew that she would at least have her younger sister's support.

In the cases of June and Deirdre (Chapters 3 and 4), where a brother was the abuser, the parents estranged themselves from their son.

In our society many people have a difficult time with their "negative" emotions—anger, sadness, grief, regret, shame, and guilt. When an adolescent or adult discloses her childhood sexual abuse to her family, these feelings factor into each family member's reaction to her; some or all of them may find themselves at a loss for ways to handle the situation. There are very few cases of happy endings for the entire family when the abuse is incestuous.

When the abuser is outside of the family, is inaccessible, or is deceased, the family's reactions tend to be more supportive of the survivor and the family more united over the issue. However, other factors may influence their response. For example, sometimes the survivor's history of acting out has caused some family members to disapprove of her, and she winds up facing a barrage of comments like

"When are you going to get over it?"

"Enough drama about something that happened twelve years ago."

"You can't use that as an excuse for everything you've done wrong."

and many other similarly unsupportive comments.

But families do not like to see other family members damaged or in pain as a result of past (or present) harm. Because it is painful to think about it, they may choose not to. Unfortunately, if they deny their own heartbreak over this and encourage the survivor to "try to forget about it," they may only compound her anger or self-hatred.

Family, friends, lovers, and spouses need to understand how important it is to acknowledge the grief and pain that come from sexual abuse. Adult survivors of childhood sexual abuse recover more successfully when family members, especially parents, use their heartbreak to be supportive, listen to them, and don't try to rush them into pretending to recover. When disclosure goes well, "going public" will be found to have been worth the risk.

Abuse survivors face different levels of denial, resistance, and rejection when they "go public," bringing the truth of their childhoods to family members who do not want to hear or accept the bad news. As we have seen, some families are receptive and supportive, which helps significantly in recovery. But it takes courage to come forward, and the results of confronting the abuser and disclosing to other family members vary widely.

33

Adolescent Date Rape

In this book we are focusing primarily on abuse that first occurs in childhood, prior to adolescence. However, there is no cutoff point after which the abused person is immune from the effects of trauma or is not at risk for developing a personality disorder. Because date rape is a significant phenomenon today, it behooves us to discuss it and give examples. Though the emphasis is on date rape occurring in adolescence, much of this material applies to date rape in adult women as well.

DATE RAPE NOT PRECEDED BY CHILDHOOD SEXUAL ABUSE

Sexual abuse during adolescence forms part of the spectrum of sexual discrimination, unwanted sexual attention, and sexual abuse that children and women experience their whole lives. The key difference between prepubescent (preteen) and postpubescent (teenage) girls is that most teenagers have had some sexual experience short of intercourse—many have experienced intercourse as well—whereas most preteens have not had any sexual experience. Childhood is the time in life when the greatest part of physical and emotional development takes place, so the slightest crossing of physical sexual boundaries can cause a child great damage (as we have seen in earlier chapters).

For teenagers, because of their familiarity with at least some sexual activity, the sexual abuse that will do the most damage to their still-developing personalities and brains—especially when accompanied by threats and brutality, which promote fear and terror—is rape. In addition, people who experience rape for the first time as adolescents usually have some protection from its negative effects due to their years of healthy, preassault development, which adolescents abused as children do not have. Nevertheless, abuse first occurring during adolescence must be taken as seriously as childhood rape and molestation, because adolescence is a time when much of future development is still available for revision and change, and abuse during adolescence can still create lifelong impairment.

Adolescent girls age twelve to sixteen usually have great difficulty revealing date rape. This is especially true if the girl is romantically involved with the rapist and prior to the rape they "made out" or sexually "fooled around" short of intercourse. When the rape occurs, she may try to rationalize her distress by accepting rape as part of an intimate relationship. The person who coerced her, forced her, or overpowered her into submitting to rape usually says something afterward like, "We just went a little further. What's the big deal?"

The girl may feel very strongly that moving from touching and being touched to being penetrated by a penis is a profound step further, but she worries that others may agree with the boy or man, that unwanted intercourse, often virginal intercourse, was just a step further than behavior she had consented to earlier. She is afraid that she will be accused of "being a tease" by leading him to "the point of no return," and therefore that she "deserved it." Mickie's case is an example of this experience.

Mickie   As one sixteen-year-old patient of mine, Mickie, tentatively put it at the beginning of her session, "I think I've been raped." She had difficulty in deciding whether or not she was enti-tled to call herself a rape victim, even though she was visibly upset by the experience. I asked her to describe what had happened.

"I had a blind date with a guy from a college town nearby, and he brought his friend along. I thought that he, or now they, were going to take me out for dinner. Instead they said it would be cool if we fooled around first. I didn't really know him, but he was hot looking so I agreed and said, "Okay, but nothing too serious since I don't know you." My blind date produced a bottle of vodka and we had some while his friend stayed in the other room. I'm a cheap high because I don't drink much. One thing led to another and I was naked and hardly self-conscious about the 'minor' penetrations and fondling between us. Then his friend appeared. I was pretty tipsy and made a mild protest. His friend grabbed my wrists and pulled my arms over my head. Then he held me down and entered me. When he was finished, they swapped positions and my date 'did' me.

"Then they told me to get dressed and we could all go out to din-ner, which we did. I think it didn't hit me. I didn't cry or anything. I even ate my dinner. Then I felt the nausea, went to the ladies' room and threw up and cried for a long time. When I came out they asked me what took so long. I told them the food didn't agree with me. They didn't notice my puffy eyes or swollen lips. They took me home and dropped me off, and my 'date' even had the nerve to call me the next day to chat."

"When did this happen?"

"Last week."

"Why didn't you tell anyone?"

"You were on vacation."

"I'm the only person you could tell?"

"I needed to figure out what to call it before I told anyone else. I couldn't do that with my parents or friends."

"How did you feel about what happened?"

"The way I felt when I was throwing up in the ladies' room—disgusting." She had an expression of shame on her face.

She needed validation despite how glaringly obvious it was that her experience was rape. Waiting a minute for my own anger at the perpetrators to subside, I said, "You've been raped."

She started to cry her saved-up tears. When she was finished she said, "But you can't tell my parents."

"How old were these boys or men?"

"They're both twenty-three."

"Mickie, under the law, I'm a mandated reporter and you're a minor."

"What does that mean?"

"It means if I don't notify the police, legally I become a coconspirator in this multiple rape."

"You make it sound like I've been gang-raped."

"You have."

"But my parents will have a fit," she protested.

"Maybe we'll tell them here, and then notify the police."

She seemed relieved.

I made a call to her father and told him that I needed to meet with him and his wife within twenty-four hours. He was worried but he agreed.

When Mickie's parents were told what had happened, they became upset, and although they were disappointed with Mickie's judgment, they agreed to go to their local police and file a complaint. The police sergeant notified me that the incident had been reported and would be investigated.

Some of Mickie's friends were supportive, while others blamed her for it. Viewing herself as suspect by other girls, Mickie initially fought back but then drifted toward promiscuous behavior and the appearance of being "easy": she behaved more hostilely and flamboyantly toward other girls, especially those who blamed her, whose boyfriends she threatened to romance. Mickie felt devalued and was experiencing a delayed reaction to the trauma of rape. This included developing defense mechanisms of denial and trying to minimize the impact this frightening and humiliating experience had had on her.

After reporting her social status and behavior to me she declared, "I don't really care what those girls think. I might even fool around with some of their boyfriends."

"Won't that make their accusations look legitimate? Perhaps it might also cause other boys to view you as a target."

"I can take care of myself—and the next guy who tries to rape me will get a good kick in the nuts."

"Rather than let the direction you're going in gain momentum, maybe you should pause and take stock of what you lost as a result of the rapes."

After a silence she became teary, "So what else should I do? They call me a whore."

"How about retreating from the dating scene for a while so this can cool down, rather than heat up until you get burned even more?"

"But I'm angry. I don't want to give in."

"How do you want this to turn out?"

"Okay . . . okay, I'm becoming someone else and maybe that's not so good."

Mickie's adolescent experience with rape may still develop into post-traumatic stress disorder. If we keep working on it, hopefully we can contain it as an "organized" memory in the hippocampus, preventing it from spilling over into the disorganized part of her brain, the amygdala. When an adolescent has the opportunity to learn to use her conscious mind to interpret her feelings, she is creating a valuable instrument for developing and maintaining emotional health in her future.

Mickie chose to disclose her date rape and struggled with the consequences of the negative reactions of others. Moira, our second example of date rape, chose to keep her date rape secret and suffered the negative legacy of keeping toxic secrets.

Moira Moira referred herself to therapy at the age of twenty-nine for self-cutting although after a few sessions she indicated that she was also an alcoholic. She had started drinking heavily at age fourteen after being raped by a nineteen-year-old boyfriend who was part of her drinking crowd. He had raped her several times, making threats that he would kill her family if she told anyone. She debated whether her tough, bad-tempered, alcoholic father could stop him and decided it was not worth the gamble. She continued to drink, but managed to get good grades in school even while drunk, and went off to a good college, where her drinking no longer stood out against a background of the widespread campus drinking scene. Then in her early twenties her drinking had cost her a serious boyfriend and a good job with a future. Now she was drinking nearly a liter of vodka a day, which only made her feel worse about herself.

Moira understood her motives for drinking, which she spoke about articulately: "I guess the alcohol initially dimmed the memory of the rapes and my powerlessness to do anything about them, and this spread to a feeling of general powerlessness to do anything about anything."

On some days, however, she came to sessions drunk; her speech was coherent but rambling, and I chided her for undermining therapy. When it became apparent that her drinking was unchanged, we arranged to admit her to the alcoholic abuse "detox" unit of a psychiatric hospital, where she remained for three months. Part of the hospital program was joining the Alcoholics Anonymous group on the hospital grounds. She continued attending AA meetings for years after her discharge from the inpatient program. Once sober, her therapy became productive and she was able to face the events that had kept her drunk for fifteen years.

DATE RAPE COMPLICATED BY CHILDHOOD SEXUAL ABUSE

Adolescent date rape can elicit criticism and suspicion of the person raped, especially from those who are not close enough to her to hear the whole story and do not have a trusting relationship with her. The criticism is a form of "blaming the victim" where strangers and acquaintances in the high school or college community look askance at the claim of rape, as they did in Mickie's story. Comments suggesting she was initially provocative and/or made foolish judgments that led to the unwanted intercourse are more frequent than sympathy for her. This is part of the risk of going public, which creates such anxiety in girls. Many girls deal with their own anxiety at hearing about someone else getting raped by telling themselves that it could not happen to them because they are different in some way from the victim. To solidify this difference they blame the raped girl for what happened to her, and she ends up blaming herself for an act of violence perpetrated by someone else. As a result, a high percentage of date rapes go unreported.

When date rape, either adolescent or adult, occurs to the same woman several times, her credibility nearly disappears. Others assume she is either lying or exaggerating what they believe to have been consensual sex.

A woman who falls into this category—experiencing multiple instances of date rape—often was molested as a child and is still living with "the forever factor": she believes she will be abused in adulthood just as she was in childhood. And just as she was helpless to control the time or frequency of the abuse when she was young, so she believes herself to be helpless now. Her combined feelings of helplessness and resignation produce in her an inadequate ability to sense danger in social situations, specifically the danger of sexual attack. Her sense of caution is greatly reduced since caution was seen as irrelevant to protecting her as a child. She may have an encounter with a man under risky circumstances: it may occur in a solitary location or "bad" neighborhood, and she may be seemingly unaware of his appearance or style—slick, overly warm, shifty, or age-inappropriate (especially if he is much older than she is).

Consciously, the girl or woman is looking to attract a male with seemingly normal desires. She wishes for an outcome that will lead to an ongoing relationship or at least a pleasant or mildly romantic encounter. Unconsciously, a woman molested or raped as a child may have a number of other motives.

One unconscious motive is to set up tests with successive men to see if the man will resist forcing himself on her—even if he has the opportunity of total privacy and she is dressed provocatively. A sexually aggressive man will likely fail these tests and rape her.

If the frequency of her childhood abuse was high, if the events occurred over a long time, and if they were perpetrated by an older male in her family, then another unconscious motive—the most difficult for those unfamiliar with child abuse to understand—is likely present: the compulsion to repeat a painful experience she consciously hates but unconsciously has adjusted to. Because the unconscious mind seeks out what is familiar, repetitions of situations that lead to rape may occur without conscious knowledge. We would have to call this *symptomatic rape* because, like self-mutilation, it is symptomatic of the original childhood abuse. Symptomatic rape (as opposed to nonsymptomatic rape) is one of the most extreme examples of self-debasement that childhood sexual abuse can spawn.

Allowing certain characteristic forms of mistreatment—such as teasing, embarrassing, humiliating, and battering behaviors—to be directed against oneself are forms of what we might call *consensual demoralization*. The significance of consensual demoralization is that, even though it is milder and less dramatic than symptomatic rape, the woman is nevertheless still unconsciously putting herself in situations where rape is likely to be the next step.

Regardless of the woman's conscious or unconscious motives, rape is still rape. As a society we must not lessen our condemnation of the rapist because of his victim's background. The rapist often uses the "pseudo-consensual sex" argument in court when he protests, "But she really wanted it!" If she "really wanted it," he would have sensed it and then she would have held little interest for him, since most rapists require the woman's fear in order to become aroused. It is important when discussing date rape not to "try the victim" in our minds. To do so risks approving of rape.

Prevention of date rape is a vital topic for discussion and teaching, both in school and at home. It is important to focus on key issues, such as the use of alcohol and drugs in the company of boys or men who are not well known to a young woman, for these factors increase the danger of date rape.

34

Combating Body Memories
with the Mind

Blaming the allure of her body, or parts of her body, for her ongoing sexual abuse is sometimes a child's way of explaining to herself why these events are happening. This blame of the body can become hidden from consciousness from the time the abuse ends (usually by age twelve). Nevertheless, body pains (sometimes referred to as "body memories") are often expressions that reside in the amygdala, where anxiety and tension remaining from past abuse are stored.

MINIMIZING AWARENESS OF SEX-RELATED BODY PARTS

Sometimes these expressions are experienced as actual pain, spasms, and contractions. In other cases they may be converted to thoughts of revulsion about breasts, the vagina, and the area around the vagina including the pubic hair. More than one young woman explained to me that she cut and bleached that hair to minimize her awareness of the organ in its center. Victims of childhood sexual abuse often maintain ignorance, by choice, about the structure and functions of organs related to the abuse they experienced. They cannot visualize the appearance or purposes of the vagina and minimize visual and tactile involvement when feminine hygiene is necessary. They are ashamed of the vagina, calling it "unclean" or "filthy."

The same avoidance exists verbally. Questions are not asked about these areas and discussions involving them are considered repulsive and so are avoided. Combating nerve impulses from the conscious mind by talking with the patient about the trauma-causing events weakens the power of these impulses to cause involuntary bodily reactions. One of the goals of therapy with such a patient is to put in perspective the terrifying notions she has about her body.

One mother of a teenage patient requested that I answer "girl" questions for her daughter, questions my patient had been asking her mother. When I asked her why she, as a woman and mother, could not answer these questions, she explained to me that even though she had been pregnant and had given birth to two children, she "had no idea what was down there or how it worked." The mother was forty-four years old and had made intimations of "disagreeable things that happened" in her childhood. It is clear that victims of child sexual abuse do not simply outgrow the damage it has done to them.

At some point in therapy the body needs to come up for discussion. This is one way of increasing confidence and desensitizing the victim to bodily fears and self-hatred. It also helps her achieve greater safety and develop a sense of confidence with her femininity.

An example of this process is Christy, the youngest patient presented in this book.

CHRISTY: RECOVERING FROM FEAR OF HER BODY

For example, several years ago an eleven-year-old, Christy, was referred to me for cutting. Her story gives us a condensed look at the damage that usually develops unconsciously over time in adult women who have been molested as children.

Christy was short for her age, had curly blond hair held close to her part by pink barrettes—all of which made her look younger than her age, more like a nine-year-old. In contrast to her appearance she had a deep, foghorn-like voice. She spoke little and responded to questions with "yes," "no," or just nods and head-shakes. I suggested that some day she would be able to talk so much during her sessions that I probably would not be able to get a word in edgewise. She cocked her head slightly to one side skeptically and said nothing.

During the next several months she did begin to talk. She explained that she was ignored by most of her classmates because she looked younger and was not ready to talk about boys yet. She had started to cut herself with her father's double-bladed safety razor. She had many one-inch pairs of shallow, parallel cuts on her left forearm. About the cutting she said, "It just makes me feel better for a while." She also said that she did well with her schoolwork, but in school "only the losers would be my friends."

She talked about her sister's social success and this led her to describe a boy in the eighth grade—Christy was in the sixth—who said he would be her friend if she let him touch her under her panties. She stared down at the floor when describing this and said that whatever he was doing hurt, but that she was afraid to complain and lose the only friend she had. One day she felt pain while urinating and told him he could not touch her anymore. He stopped talking to her.

She was ashamed and could not tell anyone, so she tried to forget the half-dozen episodes of "being poked," as she called it. "I hope he didn't break anything down there," she commented. I told her that she could visit a female doctor who would give her a brief examination appropriate to her age and reassure her about her developing body. Christy liked the idea of seeing a woman doctor, but something else was bothering her.

She voiced objections about the way her mother dressed her and expressed strong feelings about her appearance. "Look at me, I'm eleven years old, my hair is in barrettes and bangs which come down to my glasses. Even though I picked them out, they're too small—these wire frames make me look bug-eyed to boot. You know, when that boy reached under my underpants, my worst fear was that he would see them, with bluebirds and lollypops, baby panties. So I let him touch me and put his finger in a place that we learned in school was wrong, which made me bad, and that was the only way I could have a friend."

"Well, I can certainly understand how much you wanted a friend. And I think you're punishing yourself even though you didn't do anything wrong. I think that boy took advantage of your loneliness."

For the first time since we met, Christy started to cry. "So you don't think I'm bad?"

"No, I don't."

"Thank you." She blew her nose and went on. "So what am I going to do about making real friends, being that I look like the biggest nerd in the world?"

I suggested that she might talk to her mother about buying her clothes that were more like those of her classmates and doing her hair in a more grown-up style. She was worried her mother would not listen to her, so I volunteered to talk to her mother on her behalf. She was happy to have support for these requests, and within two weeks she came into the office dressed more like an early teen than a nine-year-old. She was proud of her new hairdo as well.

She sat down and stated to me, "Remember the day you said to me that one day you might not get a word in edgewise?"

"Yes, is this the day?"

"Well, I need to ask some embarrassing questions. I tried to ask my mom, but she said I was too young and I could ask some other time."

"Okay—shoot."

At this point Christy asked me about how girls are supposed to get rid of their underarm hair. Since she had cut herself with safety razors, I "prescribed" a lady's electric razor.

"Okay, good, but I'm scared about buying a bra, and using a tam-

pon, and wearing a bathing suit when I don't know how to make my
bikini line look right!" Once again she was crying. "The other girls
are fine with all of that stuff, but I feel like I'm not supposed to
touch myself down there because of, you know, what that boy did
to me."

"I see. This boy not only hurt you physically; he also made you
feel scared of your own body."

"Yeah! Is that weird?"

"No, it's a normal response to what happened. I'm going to call
your doctor and ask her to explain menstruation to you, including
everything you need to know. But I can assure you right now that
there's no part of your body that's wrong or bad for you to touch."

Christy's molestation had created an emotional conflict about
taking care of her body. Earlier mention was made of the lack of
context abused children suffer from, which often results in hatred
and blame of their bodies. In this case, as a result of being
molested, Christy was *afraid* of her body. She needed feminine
information about her body and how to take care of it. Without that
information she felt inferior, behaved shyly, and was ashamed of
her ignorance. Eventually she became ready to integrate that information and requested it. Christy needed to disclose her abuse but
was uncomfortable in talking about her female body.

Christy's mother, perhaps because of her own bad feelings about
her daughter's abuse, had not been comfortable with these important topics and had brushed off her daughter's questions. Once
Christy found a trusted adult who would treat her need for information seriously, her entire demeanor changed and she became
more confident. Additionally, puberty can be a time for accelerated
change in psychotherapy, since it is an impressionable age when
much of the personality, especially with regard to sexual identity, is
open to change.

The rapidity of Christy's change (which included giving up cutting as well) was a result of information directly related to her sexual development, especially menstruation. This information,
provided by the gynecologist, removed the mystery this area of her

body represented at the time of her molestation. Up to this point, the abusive boy had been more familiar with her genitals than she was.

Parents and therapists can help molested children and teens by giving them factual information about the female body and its development when they are ready to integrate it. Repeated discussions will reduce the negative intensity they associate with their anatomy.

The same can be said for psychotherapy with women who indicate that feminine parts of their body are off-limits for discussion or even thought. Each time the subject is revisited, discussion reduces tension and trauma to some degree.

35

To the Sexually Abused Reader: Getting the Help You Need

Do you recognize yourself in parts of this book? Perhaps you have no conscious memories of sexual abuse from childhood. Nevertheless, ask yourself: can you feel some of the feelings that survivors of childhood sexual abuse have expressed or identify with some of their behaviors? Or perhaps you do have memories of experiences you think might—or definitely do—qualify as sexual abuse. Have you kept these to yourself, telling no one? Or did you try telling them to others—friends, family members, teachers— when you were young, with unwanted results? Are you in therapy but have not told your therapist about the abuse, or talked about it in therapy but it has not helped?

FROM VICTIM TO SURVIVOR

If the answer to some or all of these questions is yes, then you are having trouble with your identity. For now, you identify as "victim." This does not mean you are immoral, filthy, evil, a coward, a slut, or a whore. It means that another person—someone who was wrong in using you—abused you. That person, not you, is the one who perpetrated an immoral action or actions by hurting you and leaving you with these bad feelings about yourself.

You are not hopelessly doomed to feel like this, but you will need help to overcome this most painful experience. Recovery can begin in many ways; the first step may be telling a friend or lover, writing down a dream, or calling a clinic or counseling center. Your biggest struggle is shame. Even when you talk about the abuse, it is important not to simply *report* it, without emotion, which you may want to do to separate the words from your feelings. You have to hear yourself say it, feel yourself say it. That will change you: You will have proclaimed who you are. You will no longer be in hiding, disguised and trapped behind a false façade that keeps shame alive.

The first person you talk to about the abuse may not be helpful. Do not give up. Keep looking for that someone who will feel right—whether it is a therapist or another helpful adult. The dialogue between you and this person must become powerful enough to drown out the negative thoughts you have about yourself, to reduce the need to hide in dissociation, and eventually to give you the strength to stare down the flashbacks. Helpful dialogue should make you want to take good care of your body. Such dialogue will take years in order to compensate for the "stolen years"—during which the abuse was a secret that kept you alone.

In addition to talking privately with a therapist or counselor, other resources are available. There are organizations that provide support groups for people who have been sexually abused. Being in these groups teaches you that you are not alone—there are others like you. You learn that it is not a disgrace to have been abused. Moreover you can share with others the disgraceful behaviors of your perpetrators and the painful feelings and thoughts that affect your life. Support groups are a good adjunct to therapy and can also serve as an introduction to therapy. A number of books have been written about survivors of both childhood and adulthood sexual abuse; some are autobiographies. We urge you to marshal your courage and determination to use all of these resources before the past does more damage to your present and future. Your goal is to remove the mark your perpetrators have left on your life.

Much of what is written addresses the task of moving from "victim" to "survivor." Everyone who works for the recovery of people who have experienced childhood sexual abuse agrees on the necessity of that transformation. This process takes time and faith in yourself. You will experience—if you are not already doing so—a struggle within yourself between old, habitual feelings, thoughts, and reactions and new ones you will try to build. Recovery involves consciously arguing with your past as you work to build a perspective on when it is necessary to protect yourself, and when it is appropriate to be vulnerable.

In all analytic, interpretive "talk therapy" the goal is to bring the unconscious impulses that drive you to think, feel, and act in certain ways out of your unconscious and into your conscious mind. This will give you choices so that you are not compelled to react to a given situation. Neurologically, that means you are using a part of your cortex called the *forebrain*, the last part of the brain to mature, instead of your amygdala, the more-primitive, less-organized part of the brain that generates impulsive, rather than well-thought-out solutions. When trauma is dominating your memory, you are deprived of the use of your "orderly" memory (located in a part of the brain called the hippocampus). This struggle—to identify what is trauma, how it affects you, and finally to weaken its hold over you with thoughts and words shared aloud with a trusted person—is what will stop your past from stealing your emotional freedom in the "now" and being a thief of your tomorrows. The first challenge is to find that trustworthy, knowledgeable person whom you are willing to speak these thoughts with. Having found this person, your second task is to use him or her as your ally in recovery, to treat this person as someone who can validate you with reflection and support. Together you can minimize the power of the past and achieve a major part of the trauma-reducing process.

FINDING AND TESTING A GOOD-ENOUGH THERAPIST

Looking for the therapist who is good enough means finding someone who can help you because he or she has the necessary personality qualities and skills to do so. However, looking for the *perfect* therapist will set you up for unending mistrust and suspicion; it will keep you stuck at step one, selecting a therapist. This does not mean you need to choose someone who has mediocre skills, who does not seem knowledgeable about your kinds of problems, or who is not interested in you in an appropriate, caring way. What it does mean is that the first struggle is with yourself, between the part of you that never wants to trust anyone because you are afraid there is a fool—or worse, a perpetrator—lurking beneath the surface of every therapist's exterior presentation, and the part of you hoping against hope to find a therapist who is neither fool nor potential abuser. Here is where using the decision-making part of you, your cortex as opposed to your impulsive amygdala, is important. If you can construct an ongoing sense of appraisal and work at being fair in your judgments, you can protect yourself from someone who would harm you or (more likely) just waste your time.

Study the therapist to see whether there is any resemblance to the predators in your life. If not, then consider giving the therapist a chance. Observe how the therapist's personality and treatment "unfold" so you can decide whether you want to risk being vulnerable during therapy sessions in exchange for reducing your sense of danger, both in therapy and elsewhere in your life.

Regarding therapy as such a trade-off at the beginning may allow you to tolerate the discomfort of early sessions until you get to a point where you can see the development of an attachment or dependency as being something that would help you. This will take time, given the time that has passed and shaped your development since your first assault. Your appraisal must then include whether or not you like the therapist, the therapist is consistent with you, and he or she seems likely to be reliable over the long period of time this therapy will take. Other character traits to look for in a therapist are confidence, warmth, and knowledge about childhood sexual abuse and trauma. The therapist's attitude should communicate interest and enthusiasm for his or her work.

Testing the therapist is important to reassure yourself that you are not walking on eggshells or having to withhold experiences and thoughts because you do not have faith in the therapist to cope adequately with them. If the therapist finds your thoughts unacceptable, reacts with shock or revulsion to what you share, or is critical of you for how you have coped, this therapeutic relationship will not be productive. If the therapist is accepting and demonstrates a comfortable curiosity that helps you open up, these are good signs.

Testing your therapist by "acting out"—doing or saying things that are provocative or argumentative—is part of normal transference within therapy. When the acting out becomes the major theme of the therapy, you are creating a relationship that is symptomatic of the same defensive behaviors that have sabotaged other relationships in your life. At some point the therapist may feel that the treatment is not productive: he or she will become less effective and may even seem less interested.

When this happens, difficult questions arise: Is your therapist too limited? Or have you stretched beyond your therapist's ability to tolerate being tested relentlessly? Therapy requires a suitable match between your needs and your therapist's skills. If numerous therapists have failed your "acting out" test, then you, like any perspective patient, may have to rethink your strategy. Your acting out may be an unconscious way to "get even" with your perpetrators and not a wholehearted desire to find a trustworthy therapist. If you feel stuck in the acting-out stage, you will need a powerful, patient therapist who can recognize and cope with this to help you move on to the next stage.

USING YOUR THERAPEUTIC ALLIANCE

Once trust is developed, you can use your new sense of safety with your therapist to create healthy change. Being confronted about your behaviors by him or her, which you once might have experienced as an attack, can now be used as an opportunity to rethink your ideas about yourself. This process of reexamining your assumptions, repeated over time, helps you feel better about yourself. You can begin to risk social closeness with others, no longer fearing that they will see in you negative traits that you have always assumed were a part of you.

As therapy progresses and you develop more faith in yourself—even being able to laugh at yourself in a way that is not sarcastic and does not put you down—you are on the road to undoing the damage to your feelings and personality that your abuser put into motion years ago.

DEVELOPING A NEW VOICE

For some survivors of childhood sexual abuse, it is helpful not only to feel free to discuss new areas of present and past experience but also to say aloud words that used to be unthinkable. In Cassie's case, for example, using the word "fucking" empowered her to express her objections to her family's formality, gave her satisfaction as if she were accusing her father, and greatly reduced her feelings of being victimized.

Support groups are helpful in this regard. They implicitly allow their members to say previously prohibited words and phrases (which may differ for each member). These include what many consider "curse words," which members are free to use and discuss. Also, speaking aloud the clinical terms used for the sex organs—body parts that before could never be named aloud and in many cases not even thought about—brings a new sense of ownership of their own bodies and validation of their experiences and feelings.

These groups also allow members to accuse their abusers (who of course are absent) with total freedom. "Telling on" the perpetrators—whether to a therapist in individual therapy, or to members of a group in group therapy or a support group—is an important part of your recovery. Doing so will reduce your feelings of being an outcast and blameworthy, and it will help you to put the events in perspective.

Combining the power of a support group and individual psychotherapy can bring you into healing conversations that will gradually remove the pain, terror, and shame of the events and acts committed against you, which you may have kept hidden and repressed for years.

Afterword

I t is hard to overestimate the destructiveness of childhood sexual abuse. The perpetrator is looking for erotic stimulation derived from exerting power over a helpless child in order to satisfy his weak sense of masculinity. In doing so he destroys much of her future, stealing her tomorrows.

As members of the public, we should not lessen our resolve to bring past perpetrators to justice. They do not get over their desire to molest or rape children as they age—most of them are still committing these acts well into their sixties. This is not surprising: If rape is an expression of the rapist's need to exercise sadistic power, this need, it might be argued, increases with age as the abuser becomes older and physically weaker, requiring in turn a smaller, weaker victim. Among types of crimes, sex crimes are widely acknowledged to have the greatest rate of recidivism and those involving children a higher rate still: according to a study published by the Center for Sex Offender Management, "child molesters have a higher rate of rearrest than rapists, 52% versus 39% when tracked over 25 years."[9] Many professionals who work with these criminals believe them to be incurable.

Childhood sexual abuse has been documented in most cultures throughout the world. Yet the seriousness of the damage it inflicts is often obscured by a societal anger at "the bully" who hurts and frightens the child. We need to understand that the abuse has lifelong effects, that those who have suffered abuse cannot simply brush it aside and move on. The specific day-by-day power of the abusive experiences and their ability to rob the developing person of a healthy future have not been fully recognized by the public. It is my hope that they will become common knowledge and used to increase prevention.

Acknowledgments

We would like to thank Jill Bialosky, our editor at W. W. Norton, for her encouragement to write this book and for coordinating the team at Norton throughout the process. Special thanks to Evan Carver for his fastidiousness and hard work as our assistant editor. His gift for organization helped bring this book to fruition. Evan was continuously attentive to the book's development at every stage.

We would also like to thank the pre- and postdoctoral psychology students at SUNY Purchase College for their research assistance under the able leadership of Dr. Shanaz Moudud.

Thanks to Susan Middleton for her valuable help as a copy editor.

Finally, we thank our literary agent, Jake Elwell, for his constant support and communication as both agent and friend.

Notes

1. Child Welfare Information Gateway, U.S. Department of Health and Human Services, www.childwelfare.gov. National Institute of Mental Health, www.nimh.nih.gov.

2. D. K. Beebe et al., "Prevalence of Sexual Assault Among Women Patients Seen in Family Practice Clinics," *Family Practice Research Journal* (1994), vol. 14, no. 3, pp. 223–28.

3. Tracy J. Jarvis et al., "Childhood Sexual Abuse and Substance Use," *Addiction* (1998), vol. 93, no. 6, pp. 865–75. Quote is from p. 865.

4. John N. Briere and Diana M. Elliot, "Immediate and Long-term Impacts of Child Sexual Abuse," *The Future of Children* (1994), vol. 4, no. 2, p. 60.

5. National Crime Victims Research and Treatment Center, Department of Psychiatry, Medical University of South Carolina (1992), www.ncvc.org.

6. Jarvis et al., p. 872.

7. *DSM IV [Diagnostic and Statistical Manual of Mental Disorders*, 4th ed.] (American Psychiatric Association, Washington, DC, 1994), p. 543.

8. L. E. O'Kelly and L. C. Steckle, "A Note on Long-Enduring Emotional Response in the Rat," *Journal of Psychology* (1938), vol. 8, pp. 125–31.

9. Center for Sex Offender Management (CSOM), *Recidivism of Sex Offenders,* May 1, 2001, www.sexoffender.com/sorecidivism_review.html.

Additional Resources

BOOKS

Angelou, Maya (1969). *I Know Why the Caged Bird Sings*. New York: Bantam Books.

Courtois, C. A. (1988). *Healing the Incest Wound: Adult Survivors in Therapy*. New York: W. W. Norton & Company.

Gil, E. (1992). *Outgrowing the Pain Together: A Book for Spouses and Partners of Adults Abused as Children*. New York: Dell Publishing.

Graber, K. (1991). *Ghosts in the Bedroom: A Guide for Partners of Incest Survivors*. Deerfield Beach, FL: Health Communications.

Hunter, M. (1992). *Joyous Sexuality*. Lanham, MD: Lexington Books.

Levine, P. A. (1997). *Waking the Tiger: Healing Trauma*. Berkeley, CA: North Atlantic Books.

Maltz, W. (1991) *The Sexual Healing Journey: A Guide for Survivors of Sexual Abuse*. New York: HarperCollins.

Muller, W. (1996). *How, Then, Shall We Live?* New York: Bantam Books.

Pennebaker, J. W. (2004). *Writing to Heal: A Guided Journal for Recovering from Trauma and Emotional Upheaval*. Oakland, CA: New Harbinger Publications.

Rothschild, B. (2000). *The Body Remembers: The Psychophysiology of Trauma and Trauma Treatment*. New York: W. W. Norton & Company.

RECOMMENDED WEB SITES

An extensive number of Web sites pertain to trauma, healing, and prevention. Some are government sponsored while others are created by charitable organizations. Most have links to related sites and reading lists. Here are some we found pertinent to our topic:

- www.omnibuswellness.org (the Web site of Melissa Bradley) has a reading list as well as available services.

- www.advocateweb.com is designed primarily for victims of sexual abuse by a therapist and other professionals, but it is a comprehensive site for all types of abuse.

- www.rainn.org (Rape, Abuse, and Incest National Network) has a twenty-four-hour hotline.

- www.trauma-pages.com provides free access to treatment resources and research.

- www.child-abuse.com (Child Abuse Prevention Network).

- www.stopitnow.org gives ways to prevent child sexual abuse.

- www.aasect.org (American Association of Sex Educators, Counselors and Therapists) provides a list of certified sex therapists in your area.

- www.siawso.org (Survivors of Incest Anonymous, or SIA), the Web site for a Twelve Step group.

- www.ascasupport.org (Adult Survivors of Child Abuse) offers online information to assist survivors and a helpful workbook-style manual.

Index